PHYSICAL
REHABILITATION
OUTCOME
MEASURES

**Produced by a Working Group convened by
Health Services Directorate,
Health Programs and Services Branch
Health Canada
and
The Canadian Physiotherapy Association**

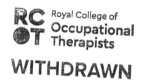

The Canadian Physiotherapy Association Health Outcomes Model illustrates the three spheres of education, practice and research as interconnected. The model acknowledges and validates all three spheres. The model promotes the concept that when and where all three spheres intersect, the result is a client-centered quality health outcome.

Physical Rehabilitation Outcome Measures

Beverley Cole

Elspeth Finch

Carolyn Gowland

Nancy Mayo

Editor, John Basmajian

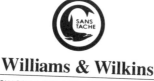

Williams & Wilkins

BALTIMORE • PHILADELPHIA • HONG KONG
LONDON • MUNICH • SYDNEY • TOKYO

A WAVERLY COMPANY

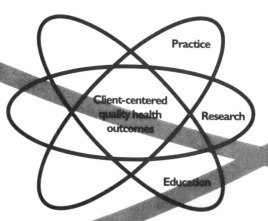

Practice

Client-centered quality health outcomes

Research

Education

Distributed worldwide (except Canada) by:
Williams & Wilkins
351 West Camden Street
Baltimore, Maryland 21201-2436, USA

Domestic		International	
Phone	(800) 638-0672	Phone	(410) 528-4223
FAX	(800) 447-8438	FAX	(410) 528-8550

In Canada copies may be purchased from:
Canadian Physiotherapy Association
890 Yonge Street, 9th Floor
Toronto, Ontario
M4W 3P4

Phone	(416) 924-5312	FAX	(416) 924-7335
	(800) 387-8679		

Published by the Canadian Physiotherapy Association in cooperation with
Health and Welfare Canada and the Canada Communications Group -
Publishing, Supply & Services Canada.

ISBN 0-683-18002-9
Printed in CANADA

FOREWORD

This manual is a groundbreaking event and is a pleasure to have. It documents, for the first time, the knowledge base in outcome measures in physical rehabilitation. With the emphasis in all health care systems to demonstrate the cost effectiveness of physical rehabilitation it could not be more timely. Here is a centralized source of "powerful" information on outcome measures; powerful in the sense that it enables us to apply available measures judiciously, giving us the opportunity to appreciate their usefulness and limitations. Its clear and "user friendly" format should secure its place as a working reference for clinicians, the intended primary user.

A major strength is the template that is used to present the characteristics of each measure from administrative to scientific properties. This template enables easy retrieval of information and provides a basis for comparing measures. Where available, the information is backed by research and or references.

The variability in the psychometric properties of the measures may surprise you, as it did me. Although I suspected as much, the format and the comprehensive coverage gave me a first time look across the many measures that we use. Some measures are less well developed than others. Although we might attest to the usefulness of these less developed measures through clinical experience, we also know that personal experience is not enough. Hereto, this manual is a gold mine. The standard categories of information used to describe each measure make it easy to identify clinical studies that need to be done by clinicians and researchers.

The challenge now is to develop this document further in future editions, as new information accumulates in the research literature and critical analysis of each measure becomes possible. This manual could be the forerunner of a standard reference document in physical rehabilitation, as "Buros" Mental Measurement Yearbook is for test users in Education and Psychology.

I congratulate the Canadian Physiotherapy Association, Health Canada, the editor and others who have contributed to the development of this manual. A significant milestone in the evolution of a profession is documentation of its measures. I hope that the use of this manual goes beyond the borders of Canada to colleagues worldwide.

Carmella Gonnella Ph.D., P.T.
Professor Emerita
Department of Rehabilitation Medicine
Emory University
Former President, American Congress of
Rehabilitation Medicine

FOREWORD

It is not surprising that current physiotherapy practice, as revealed by the survey reported in this manual, involves only a limited use of outcome measures. When the Canadian National Health Research and Development Program (NHRDP) identified the paucity of adequate outcome measures as an impediment to the development of research in rehabilitation and had a special competition in 1987, the concept of outcome measures was also new to the research community and even though 174 letters of intent were submitted, only 11 of the 54 applications received were funded.[1] The results of these funded projects, were presented at the First National Rehabilitation Outcome Measures Conference held in Edmonton in 1991 and published in a special issue of the Canadian Journal of Public Health.[1] Then, as now, as confirmed by papers presented at the Second National Rehabilitation Research Conference: Outcome Assessments in Rehabilitation, held in Quebec City in September 1993, outcome measures related to the impairment and disability concepts were more numerous than those related to the handicap concept. Abstracts of these papers were published in a special issue of the Canadian Journal of Rehabilitation.[2] Nevertheless, clinicians and researchers alike have come a long way in a short time in recognizing the value of appropriate outcome measures, especially when used within the framework of the World Health Organization (WHO) classification relating to the consequences of injury and disease process.

This manual is an important and timely contribution to clinical and research activities in physical rehabilitation. It presents, under one cover, an overview of the WHO classification, an introduction to measurement theory that emphasizes the importance of reliability and validity as applied to outcome measures, and a compendium of the best known clinical outcome measures summarized in a format for easy reference. The template presentation of each measure summarizes its characteristics, application and psychometric properties. The writing style is clear and precise and users will find this manual easy to read and the information to be very logically organized. Clinicians, educators and researchers will appreciate the compendium of measures that will save hours of independent research to find and organize the material. I believe this manual should be a required text in physiotherapy curricula in the universities and be available in physiotherapy clinical departments. It is imperative that physiotherapists evaluate the effects of their interventions and the use of outcome measures with appropriate research designs (be it single case studies or randomized controlled trials). Proper use of outcome measures will impact on the quality and cost of rehabilitation. It is also important to remember, however, that clinical outcome measures, in general, document change over time but do not explain why the change has occurred. For example, when strength is used as an outcome measure it does not tell you if a weakness is due to poor activation of agonist muscles, to excessive coactivation of antagonist muscles or to other reasons. Thus, a word of caution; our fascination with outcome measures should not inhibit inquiry into the mechanisms underlying change, because knowledge of these mechanisms is essential to the development of rehabilitation theory and new treatment strategies.

In closing, I would like to recognize the contribution and leadership provided by physiotherapists and physicians in Hamilton and Montreal who developed at least 6 of the measures presented in this manual. I congratulate the editor, and the physiotherapy educators and researchers who were members of the Working Group: Beverley Cole, Elspeth Finch, Carolyn Gowland and Nancy Mayo for having undertaken and completed the immensely difficult task of writing and organizing this compendium of outcome measures with the financial and administrative help of Health Canada and the Canadian Physiotherapy Association. I trust that this manual will lead to future editions that will keep this compendium up to date and eventually broaden its scope to include outcome measures spanning all aspects of rehabilitation.

References

1. Canadian Journal of Public Health 1992:83: suppl.2: July/August.

2. Canadian Journal of Rehabilitation 1993: 7: fall.

Carol L. Richards, Ph.D., P.T.
Professor and Director
Physiotherapy Department
Laval University

PREFACE

This is a user-friendly manual written to promote and facilitate the use of outcome measures by clinicians in rehabilitation. It is based on feedback from a cross-sectional survey of 209 Canadian physical therapists on their use of, their concerns about, and their attitudes towards, outcome measures. Part I provides the rationale for the use of these measures as an integral part of the decision-making process in clinical practice. In Part II, the presentation of survey results yields fascinating information on the current usage of these measures and highlights the information therapists feel would facilitate their use of these measures as an integral part of clinical practice. Part III, the Heart of the Matter, provides the information clinicians requested. It is written to enhance the reader's ability to first select, then critically review, the measures that meet their needs and those of their clients. We provide a novel template design to facilitate the process. Then, using the template, we review 60 important measures for the reader in 4 major areas of practice including: adult neurological and functional activity; back and pain; cardiopulmonary; and developmental paediatrics, to ensure there is at least one measure of interest to every practitioner.

Part IV is the next step in the process, where we help the reader implement a system for outcome measurement. Using the International Classification for Impairment, Disability and Handicap framework, we show how to choose the appropriate tool based on the attribute the individual wishes to measure. The measurement of treatment outcomes of both individual and groups of clients is discussed. In Part V, we outline the challenges for readers of different backgrounds who are ready to participate in the evolution of evidence-based practice in this country .

This document is targeted first at physical therapists, especially clinicians, whose clinical decision-making abilities will be enhanced by the incorporation of valid, standardized outcome measures. It will also benefit students and other professionals who are involved in clinical decision making in physical rehabilitation. Finally this document will be of interest to managers and decision makers in rehabilitation who believe in accountability and the effective and efficient use of available human and financial resources. If this book is used as intended it will facilitate the use of outcome measures in clinical practice and consequently the evolution of the practice of rehabilitation in Canada. Ultimately it is our clients that stand to benefit most.

ACKNOWLEDGEMENTS

This document is the product of a process, a more exhaustive and time-consuming process than many of those involved envisioned at the outset. In the spring of 1991, Serge Taillon, a rehabilitation consultant from the Health Services Directorate, Health Canada, contacted the Canadian Physiotherapy Association (CPA) to identify an appropriate group of experts to review two jointly produced landmark documents.[1,2] The department was trying to determine whether these visionary documents, Toward Assessment of Quality of Care in Physiotherapy (Vol I & II), produced over 10 years earlier by leaders in the profession, should be reprinted, revised or replaced. Members of that initial group included France Hamel, Louis Tremblay, Patty Solomon, Steven Lawless, Elspeth Finch, Murray Maitland and myself. The group decided that the enormous evolution in the fields of quality management and outcome measurement made a revision impossible. However, the necessity of continued work in this area was underlined and so three group members prepared a new funding proposal to Health Canada to do just that.

The purpose of the project was to promote the use of standardized outcome measures in clinical decision-making. Funding for this project was approved and a new working group met for the first time in the late fall of 1991. Elspeth Finch and myself were joined by Angela Busch, a clinician from Edmonton interested in quality management, Carolyn Gowland, a researcher involved in the development and implementation of outcome measures, and Nancy Mayo, Ph.D. an epidemiologist from Montreal to help us conduct a survey of current practice. Judith Dowler and later Louise Bouchard joined us as the representatives from Health Canada. Although Murray Maitland was unable to join the working group and Angela Busch had to leave a short time after its inception, both were instrumental in determining the direction of the working group. The group was later joined by Dianne Parker-Taillon, and in her absence Janice Miller, as Director of Education, Practice and Research, representing the CPA.

Health Canada has provided generous support of the project from the outset. In addition, they supported the excellent work by Jacquie Barnett, Carol Kelsey, and Barbara Mazer who reviewed the measures, and that of Nancy Mayo who conducted a nation-wide survey. The Canadian Physiotherapy Association is the publisher and distributor of this document. They have generously permitted this first use of the CPA Health Outcomes Model, shown on the cover, developed by the CPA Strategic Planning Committee. In addition they provided the assistance of Giuliano Tolusso, Director of Communications and Public Affairs and Diane Charter, Managing Editor, Physiotherapy Canada.

It has been a pleasure and a privilege to work with Dr. John V. Basmajian, whose contribution to this document has far exceeded what one could ever expect from an editor. Likewise the work of our "typist" Gerry Karlovic was that of a superb administrative assistant. The document you are about to read is far more extensive than any of us imagined at the outset. It is not easy for any group to reach a consensus and produce a document of this nature. Credit is due to the members of the Working Group for the long hours they have put into its production; to the universities where they work and to their families for tolerating long hours of personal time spent. They worked not for the recognition they would expect from publication in a peer-reviewed journal, and not for monetary gain. This was a heartfelt service to their Association, to their clients and their colleagues. It will be their invaluable gift to the science of rehabilitation and evidence-based practice.

It has been an honour to work with all of you.

Beverley Cole
Chair
Working Group on Outcome Measures

CONTRIBUTORS

WORKING GROUP

Chair: Beverley Cole, MBA, MSc, BScPT, Assistant Professor, School of Occupational Therapy and Physiotherapy, McMaster University, Hamilton, Ontario.

Elspeth Finch, MHSc, BSc P & OT, Assistant Professor, School of Occupational Therapy and Physiotherapy, McMaster University, Hamilton, Ontario and Department of Physical Therapy, University of Toronto, Toronto, Ontario.

Carolyn (Kelley) Gowland, MHSc, PT, Associate Professor, School of Occupational Therapy and Physiotherapy, McMaster University, Hamilton, Ontario.

Nancy Mayo, PhD, MSc, BScPT, Assistant Professor, Department of Medicine, McGill University, Montreal, Quebec.

Louise Bouchard, MHA, BScOT, Rehabilitation Consultant, Health Services Directorate, Health Canada.

Judith Dowler, MBA, BN, Chief, Human Resources Unit, Health Services Directorate, Health Canada.

Dianne Parker-Taillon, MSc (Kin), BScPT, Director, Education, Practice and Research, Canandian Physiotherapy Association.

Janice Miller, BScPT, Acting Director, Education, Practice and Research, Canadian Physiotherapy Association.

Editor and Illustrator: John V. Basmajian, O. Ont, MD, FRCPC, FRCPS (Glasg), FACA, FSBM, FABMR, FACRM (Australia), Hon Dip (St L C), Professor Emeritus in Medicine and Anatomy, McMaster University, Hamilton, Ontario.

OUTCOME MEASURES REVIEWERS

Jacqueline (Jacquie) Barnett, MSc, BScPT
Carol Kelsey, MSc, BScPT
Barbara Mazer, MSc, BScOT

CONTENTS

C.   Cardiopulmonary Measures

D.   Developmental Measures

PART I

WHY AM I READING THIS ?

Good Question! Choose from the following:

1. It is time for clinicians to take responsibility for the selection and use of outcome measures.

2. I want to measure the effectiveness of my treatments and therapeutic procedures.

3. I want to meet the expected standards relative to measuring outcomes.

4. I'd like to have data relating to clinical outcomes for both myself and others (administrators, accrediting bodies, etc).

5. I'm one of the above groups of "others" whose bottom line looms large.

6. All of the above.

7. None of the above.

CHOICE "1" It is time for clinicians to take responsibility for the selection and use of outcome measures.

This, on second thought, is a reasonable choice, but I suppose it was expected of me because I opened this book. Give me some background facts.

Fact

(a) History is an open book. It shows that all professions that hope to advance their practices must take three giant leaps forward to achieve their goals. They must first **document the status and process of practice**, then **develop valid standards of practice**, and always they must **test the outcome** of their actions on behalf of their clients. To some extent physical therapy, both world-wide and in Canada, has made progress in the first two of these three endeavours. As professionals we must take responsibility now for the third requirement: outcome measures, i.e. valid, standardized tests of change.

(b) Along with the whole field of medical rehabilitation, physical therapists have widely accepted the **International Classification of Impairments, Disabilities, and Handicaps** developed and published in 1980 by the World Health Organization (WHO) in Geneva.[1] This manual of classification relating to the consequences of disease provided a unifying framework and integration of ideas. It summarized the application of the useful concepts and gave a usable terminology and subclassification of impairments, disabilities and handicaps. Coming when it did, it helped stimulate physical therapy to increase its earnest efforts to develop valid standards of practice based on the present state of the art and science, and it provided a conceptual model which made sense in rehabilitation.

That's a fine lecture, but it sounds like what researchers say to each other; how am I, a clinician, supposed to relate to and to use <u>outcome measures</u>?

Fact

(a) The need for standards and for measuring the consequences of impairments and their treatment was implied throughout the WHO book, but no attempt was made by the task forces and revision conferences to provide practical approaches to outcome measures. The effort to provide the "how-to" has been occurring in the past two decades in both the development of **a basic understanding of the issues**,[2-5] and **applications for general use in rehabilitation**.[6,7]

(b) The development of applications for use in rehabilitation has resulted in a number of test instruments used to rationalize the team effort as it affects humane client care, as well as an improvement of cost/benefit ratios for both individuals and payer agencies. In the past year or two, the FIM (Functional Independence Measure)[7] has become the dominant measure in North America while several other useful measures of health and disability remain in active use as well.[8,9] It seems safe to predict that the FIM will emerge as the gold standard because of the enormous research programs now testing it. This measure which is imbedded in its own database — the Uniform Data Set for Medical Rehabilitation (UDS) — provides a method for evaluating outcomes in general rehabilitation populations. However, this global approach becomes more difficult and less relevant to apply and appreciate the farther it gets from general rehabilitation populations such as stroke.

Aha! You've struck a raw nerve. I'm a clinician, and already you've slipped into "research".

Fact

Relax! This present document is not written for researchers; it is meant for clinicians who conscientiously hope to improve their practices both for individuals and for groups under their care. However, it is not a rote "how-to" book. Neither is it the final word. Hence the research-minded also have an opportunity of finding in these pages a great deal of challenge and conceptual ferment.

The ultimate goal of this document is to promote the clinical use of outcome measures to evaluate the **provision of physical therapy services** using the WHO classification as the major base. Hence **Declaration I**.

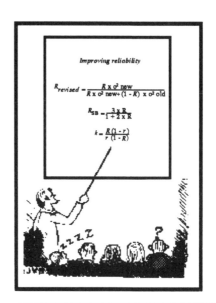

DECLARATION I

*It is hereby resolved that we – clinicians involved in physical rehabilitation – will **promote the clinical use of outcome measures to evaluate the provision of physical therapy services** using the WHO classification of Impairment, Disability and Handicap as the major base.*

OK, I've read your "declaration", but how did you arrive at it?

Fact

(a) The Working Group struggled with this and reached a consensus during 1992. They set about their preliminary tasks by reviewing available resource documents, preparing the survey (upon which Part II of this publication is based), and arranging for the preparation and issuance of this publication during 1994.

(b) The Group will persist in its efforts BY encouraging the use of the approach outlined in this book, demonstrating at every opportunity how clinicians can use the outcome measures. They will clarify how clinicians (both those who are not and those who are using some measures now) could implement the recommendations.

(c) From the start, there was agreement that generally a range of outcome measures with critical reviews should be provided that can be applied to different groups in a variety of settings. Clients should be ensured some appropriate level of outcome measurement.

I'm impressed by what you say, but surely that isn't the end of it. What will you do for me, assuming this document was a first formal step for Canadian physical therapists?

We, the Working Group, agree this is only a first step for physical therapists and all members of the rehabilitation team and leads naturally to Declaration II, below.

DECLARATION II

For the future, we, the Working Group, recommend that therapists individually and collectively make optimal use of outcome measures and. . .

1. *Recommend future directions for the use of outcome measures in clinical practice, revealing gaps and making suggestions for further work, research, revision and refinement.*

2. *For the longer term, we all should promote the use of valid outcome measures in the profession by offering a plan of implementation where possible (e.g. training workshops, teaching tools, publications, etc).*

CHOICE "2" I want to measure the effectiveness of my treatments and therapeutic procedures.

When I was first admitted to my educational program I had a marvellous vision of the profession as a healing art based firmly on the sciences. I believed that everything we would do with our clients would be beneficial. In university, I quickly realized that we are often unsure of the results of our treatments. I began to question the sequence of cause-proper treatment-effect. In my practice today these questions have taken on more importance and many remain unanswered. How will the use of outcome measures help me answer them?

Fiction

Embracing the concept of outcome measures will eliminate all your doubts and tell you once and for all which treatments to use and which ones to stop using.

Fact

You can accept the findings of researchers – and they are now becoming voluminous – that not everything we do in the name of therapy is **successful** or the **final word**. You can resolve to reduce the elements in your practice that depend heavily on the preachings of charismatic leaders. You can rely on your own ability to plan a treatment based on your findings and to test the outcome of that treatment. Common sense dictates that individual therapists must determine what procedures are truly beneficial and directly related to outcomes. Valid and standardized outcome measures can help you accomplish this in your practice. They will allow you to base future treatment on the results of your findings with similar clients.

CHOICE "3" I want to meet the expected standards relative to measuring outcomes.

I'm genuinely concerned about keeping up with the best in current practice. Certainly there is ferment for change and the use of outcome measures seems like a "sure thing" at this stage of development of practice. Maybe I could ignore the whole thing, but I don't see myself as a block to changes which will help my practice. It's more interesting to be part of the majority and it looks like there is a genuine interest in the use of outcome measures and a desire for "know how". On the other hand, I want to be sure this bandwagon is really going to help me and my clients.

Fact

One fact that we should face from the beginning is that the measurement of outcomes will not happen overnight, because it is a complex matter. This fact is evidenced by the interest of a great number of therapists in outcome measurement and the few who have a process for doing it. Much of the complexity with this topic relates to the many possible reasons for wanting to measure outcomes – the many varied environments and types of clients we are dealing with. From the survey we conducted with program managers and individual therapists we concluded that it is not a cookbook you would welcome, but rather an understanding of the issues. You are also looking for suggestions or guidelines for possible methods of implementing a system for outcome measurement that is in keeping with the goals of your clinical setting.

Fact

The National Workshop on Patient Outcome Measures[2] held "way back" in 1990 had already identified that:

- interventions are commonly not subjected to evaluation before they become common practice
- it is increasingly difficult to mount convincing arguments in favour of introducing new interventions and even maintaining many well established ones in the face of uncertainty and lack of consensus about their efficacy
- our current quality management activities are not designed to give us a clear focus of what constitutes appropriate care
- progress in outcome measurement has been impeded by assertions from health professionals that their clients are unique
- outcomes are usually defined by the provider, not the clients and caregivers. While the two may be complementary, they may not be the same
- incentives in the health care system are working against us. Funding is volume driven, not quality driven
- many health care professionals are threatened by outcome measurement.

Fact

The American Congress of Rehabilitation Medicine has recently published standards for those who use these measures. They have kindly allowed us to reprint them for you in this document. We have put them in Part III (p. 32). You will need to read them to gain a better understanding of what the expected **standards** are.

As you can see, the implementation of outcome measures in rehabilitation is evolving as different groups publish principles and methods as to how this can be done. Some additional reasons for why we are measuring outcome are given in Table 1.1.

Table 1.1: Some Purposes for Measuring Outcomes

To determine:

- The impact of an overall treatment program on an individual.

- The impact of a specific treatment approach on an individual (e.g. outcome measurement within a single case study).

- The overall impact of care on all clients within a program.

- Relative outcomes in a group of individuals in order to identify those who benefit most and least from the services provided.

- Productivity – to assess treatment outcomes in conjunction with resources used in order to assess the effectiveness and efficiency of the services provided.

- etc.

I'm beginning to see that my candid picking of choice "3" was justified. Indeed I <u>must</u> *keep up with this wave of the future, partially because it's more rewarding being part of the action, but more importantly because data are needed to aid in making rational decisions about utilization of resources.*

Can't I wait until outcome measures are developed by other professionals and then use them?

The simple answer is **NO**. Who better than ourselves to develop measures in physical rehabilitation outcomes?

CHOICE "4"   I'd like to have data relating to clinical outcomes for both myself and others (administrators, accrediting bodies, etc).

Fact

Employing the WHO classification of **IMPAIRMENT – DISABILITY – HANDICAP** (really the bed-rock of our decision making) we should be able to identify the **attribute**s of outcomes that are important – those things which we believe that rehabilitation provides to clients and which are of value – from the clients' perspective.

Fact

As clinicians, we need evidence with which to evaluate the effectiveness of our practice. In addition, we must provide others including the "payers for service" (public, government, industry) with a clear idea of what they are getting for their money.

CHOICE "5"   I'm one of the above groups of "others" whose bottom line looms large.

I've been sitting here reading all that has been said so far, but still have concerns – We already have systems in place for making funding decisions. Why are these no longer acceptable? Why should we further redirect resources away from client care to develop outcome measures and implement new systems? What's the cost of creation and development of systems for measuring outcomes? Will the use of outcome measures create an additional burden for individual clients?

Facts and Predictions

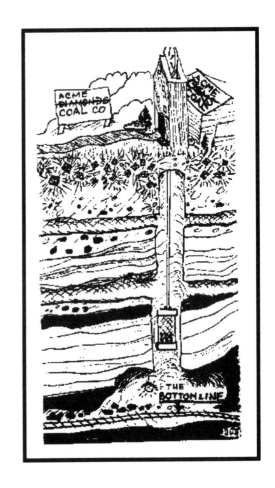

Present Status: In rehabilitation we have been so busy caring for an overwhelming number of clients that we have had little time to develop criteria for judging outcomes on the basis of objective tests. We are with the majority of health professionals in this regard. However, clinicians must rationalize current practices, improve evaluative and prognostic methods and tools, and gradually eliminate all wasteful and useless procedures. That all takes time. Only clinicians can apply these findings in practice and stimulate researchers to ask and investigate the clinically important questions.

The cost in time and money for improvement of health care (by being able to measure outcomes) is a valuable investment. Otherwise therapists would continue to employ methods that ought to be supplanted or dropped. Progress in health care depends on measurements that reflect outcomes of value to clients.

Bottom Line: Outcome measures offer great promise for identifying client needs, effectively knowing what treatment can accomplish, and allocating scarce resources. But single-minded bottom line considerations can miss the motherlode of opportunity for future progress unless the bottom line which is important to clients is included for consideration.

CHOICE "6" All of the Above.

I concede. Let me get on with Part II.

CHOICE "7" None of the Above.

My reasons are different, but perhaps the information in the next few sections will meet my needs too. Meanwhile, you haven't answered my most vexing question:

Where do I find the time?

Of course, I'd like to find out how my clients are doing, but given the existing measures in my field, I face a set of dilemmas. Do I –

a) *treat 40 clients a day (as now) using no outcome measures?*

b) *treat 30 clients a day using standardized outcome measures on the group I am most concerned about?*

c) *treat as few as 15 - 20 clients a day using some standardized outcome measures with all? ... what happens to the 20 or more clients I haven't seen that day? ... and how do I decide which 15 to 20 to treat?*

LOOK AT THE CONSEQUENCES

Answer (a)

You are already bogged down, so that is no choice at all, is it?

Answer (b)

This is a good start because you can look at the most frustrating situations. Learning how little change is occurring in the outcomes clients want can lead you to dropping some practices you doubt and finding better ways. You will end up saving time and serving the clients optimally.

Answer (c)

You will derive a great deal of practical information on what changes are occurring, in what time period, for the clients who, in your clinical judgement, are more likely to be positively affected by therapy. This will permit you to:

- decrease frequency and/or duration of treatment while producing the same or better results
- change treatment approaches and evaluate how that changes outcome

- identify those people who will benefit most from the proposed treatment

- reduce recurrence of problems by adequately evaluating prevention strategies.

- become more knowledgeable and skilled in the areas where you can have the greatest impact.

Indeed, What About the "Untreated 20"?

In this case, the great need for planning by all co-workers in a facility is essential. A real possibility exists that the 20 you "don't see" may serve as both a goal and a constant reminder of the greater need. In fact you may discover they make considerable progress.

A Shift of Mind-Set

We are looking at a profound change. We must shift away from trying to be all things to all people. We must measure outcomes and exercise rational decision making to provide logical choices that will enhance the lives of those we serve.

PART II: SURVEY

The field of medical rehabilitation has, in recent years, become increasingly focused on quality care and management. The importance of being client or customer oriented is repeatedly underlined in all areas of practice. Before writing this book, we felt it was imperative to determine the extent to which standardized measures were used by physical therapists to evaluate client outcomes. We wanted to know which factors contributed to the use of standardized outcome measures and what, in your mind, would help you most to further increase their use in your everyday practice. In this chapter, a brief description (i.e. key elements) of the methodology and the complete results of a cross-sectional survey of 209 Canadian physical therapists and directors are presented. This description underlines where you are, and what help you'd like to get to where you'd like to be. The design and information in the rest of the book is based on these results.

THE "SAMPLE"

We carried out what is known as a cross-sectional survey of 209 physical therapists and directors licensed in Canada for 1992 using a stratified, random sampling strategy, where the strata were the provinces.

A list of all licensed therapists was obtained from the provincial licensing bodies. The individuals were identified as to whether they were listed as a therapist or a director and a random sample was drawn from each group proportional to the size of the membership in each province. For most provinces the number of therapists was small enough to count and, thus, each person listed was assigned a sequential identification number and a table of random numbers was consulted to choose the identification number to be selected. For Ontario and Quebec, the number of therapists was too great and, therefore, a table of random numbers was used to select first the page number to be consulted and then the identification number that had been assigned sequentially to therapists listed on that page. This process was repeated for the directors. Ontario did not list directors separately from therapists; therefore, the list of selected individuals was sent to the main office of the Canadian Physiotherapy Association and the status of the individual was obtained subsequently from CPA.

The name and address of each person selected were entered into a computerized database management system. Each person was mailed a questionnaire along with a stamped return envelope. An attempt was made to trace individuals whose questionnaires were returned by the post office and if successful, the address was changed and questionnaire re-sent. After one month, those persons not returning questionnaires were called and reminded of the survey. If desired, the questionnaire was filled out over the phone.

The size of the sample was chosen to obtain an error rate of no more than 5%.

QUESTIONNAIRES

Two questionnaires were prepared, one for therapists and one for physical therapy directors. These questionnaires were basically similar in content but differed slightly in the phrasing of questions because we wanted therapists to respond for themselves but directors to respond for the whole department.

The questionnaire was pre-tested on a convenient sample of 120 therapists working in facilities in Montreal, Hamilton, Toronto, and Edmonton. We found in pretesting the questionnaire that therapists had not universally been exposed to the term "outcome measures" and did not know to what we were referring. Based on this, we rephrased the question in the final version to ask what tools were used to document clients' progress and offered, as one of the choices, "published measurement scales", a term which we later equated with "standardized outcome measures".

The questionnaire was designed to obtain information on the primary issue, use of standardized outcome measures. A number of secondary issues related to satisfaction and attitude toward use of measures in clinical practice, and to professional and workplace characteristics of the therapists and directors were also included.

DATA ANALYSIS

Data relating to both the preliminary and secondary issues were gathered. Therapists and directors were both asked to list all published measurement scales used. However, therapists' and directors' responses were not compared as they were responding to different questions. For therapists, the questions were related to their practice and, thus, the unit of analysis is the individual therapist. Directors, on the other hand, were responding for the department which they direct and, thus, the unit of analysis was the department which comprises more than one therapist, and a wider mix of clients according to age and diagnostic category. Therapists and directors were compared only on pattern of response and professional characteristics.

RESULTS

A total of 207 staff physical therapists and 102 physiotherapy directors were surveyed. After excluding persons who were no longer practising in Canada or on temporary leave, 176 therapists (85%) and 86 directors (84%) were eligible to participate. One hundred and forty-three therapists and 66 directors responded, yielding closely similar response rates of 81% and 77%, for therapists and directors respectively.

Analysis of the personal characteristics of the responders (Table 2.1) showed directors were more senior than therapists, as illustrated by their year of graduation; however, in comparison to therapists, significantly fewer directors had attained training beyond the level of a diploma. In those instances where the director did not fill out the questionnaire but assigned this task to another person (23% of the time), these persons were still responding for the department and not for themselves.

The majority of persons worked with a mixed group of clients comprising adults, seniors and children. Forty-five percent of therapists worked with only one type of client, mostly orthopaedic or neurological. In contrast, only 17% of departments were specialized to one type of client. Many facilities provided more than one type of service, the most common service provided was acute care (54% and 58% for therapists and directors respectively) followed by rehabilitation (47% and 48% respectively) and long-term care (32% and 35% respectively). The number of staff members working at the various facilities varied widely, ranging from less than one full-time therapist to more than 50. Most staff members (70%) were working full time.

Table 2.1: Personal Characteristics of Responding Therapists and Directors*

	Staff		Directors	
	Number	**%**	**Number**	**%**
Training				
Diploma	29	20	24	36
Bachelor's degree	106	74	37	56
Master's degree or higher	8	5	4	6
Not reported		6	1	2
Year of graduation from physical therapy				
1950-69	18	13	32	49
1970-74	17	12	6	9
1975-79	28	20	11	17
1980-84	25	18	9	14
1985-89	36	25	7	11
1990	19	13	1	12

* Multiple responses permitted

CURRENT USE OF OUTCOME MEASURES

Therapists and directors were first asked which tools were used in their department to document a client's progress in therapy. Their answers are outlined in Table 2.2. Approximately 41% of staff and 49% of directors thought that published measurement scales were being used in their departments. Therapists were then asked to list the published measurement scales used in their departments. Both therapists and directors were then asked whether they were satisfied with the way a client's progress was documented in their department. The results are also contained in Table 2.2. Only a small proportion of respondents were completely satisfied with their current method of documenting client's progress (11 therapists (8%) and 8 directors (12%)); the majority were only moderately satisfied (60% of therapists and 59% of directors), leaving another 25% to 30% either neutral or dissatisfied with their current system.

Table 2.2:   Documentation of Client Progress

	Staff		Directors	
	Number	**%**	**Number**	**%**
Tools used to document client progress				
Published measurement scales	58	41	32	49
Departmentally developed instruments only	26	18	34	52
Mechanical devices	109	76	53	80
Degree of satisfaction with current system				
Completely satisfied	11	8	8	12
Moderately satisfied	86	60	39	59
Neither satisfied nor dissatisfied	20	14	8	12
Moderately dissatisfied	22	15	9	14
Not at all satisfied	4	3	1	2
Not reported			1	2

* Multiple responses permitted

We also wanted to know if you thought the way the members of your department document a client's progress could be improved by using published measurement scales. This is the point in the questionnaire where the terminology used in the preceding sentence was first equated with standardized outcome measures. Here 82% of staff and 85% of directors felt the use of these measures would improve the documentation of a client's progress. Over 90% of therapists and 85% of directors felt that the actual monitoring of a client's progress would improve. We also wondered if you felt that the routine use of these measures would change your approach to client care. Again a larger number of therapists than directors (34% versus 24%) thought their approach to client care would change. The majority of both groups, however, either didn't know (27% and 41%) or thought that there would be no change (39% and 35%) if outcome measures were used routinely in their department.

The next logical step for us was to try to identify any barriers to the use of these measures. We asked if there was anything that prevents the members of your department from using published measurement scales to document a client's progress. We didn't use the word barriers as we didn't want to create any where they didn't exist. The majority of those answering (56% of therapists and 64% of directors) felt there were multiple factors that prevented their using these measures. These factors are listed in Table 2.3 in order of descending importance. The most frequently cited barrier was the limited knowledge of available instruments. Next in importance was not having sufficient time. Almost 38% of directors thought that available measures don't meet the needs of their clients. But a considerably smaller percentage of therapists (22%) agreed. The therapists cited that not knowing how to develop instruments was the third most significant factor preventing their use.

Table 2.3: Barriers to the Use of Standardized Outcome Measures

	Staff		Directors	
	Number	**%**	**Number**	**%**
Barriers to use of standardized outcome measures*				
None	7	5	2	3
Single barrier	56	39	22	33
Multiple barriers	80	56	42	64
Specific barriers identified*				
Limited knowledge of instruments	64	45	30	46
Time	61	43	31	47
Limited knowledge of instrument development	41	29	22	33
Don't meet need of clients	32	22	25	38
Lack of consensus on what to use	20	14	13	20
Don't know	18	13	4	6
Other	12	8	6	9
Other problems identified by respondents				
Lack of necessary equipment	5	4	2	3
Administrative barriers	2	1	3	5
Lack of knowledge of utility	2	1	1	2

* Multiple responses permitted

Finally, before we asked how we could help, we needed to know whether you thought that the use of standardized outcome measures to document a client's progress could have a <u>negative impact</u> on the practice of physical therapy in Canada. Here 15% of therapists and 24% of directors answered yes. That sounds like there are a fair number of you we'll just have to work harder to convince. The majority in both groups thought there would be no negative impact (67%, 53%) or they had no opinion (18% and 23%). We suspect concerned onlookers might be quite encouraged by these statistics!

Finally, we were getting to our raison d'être. We asked you "would you be interested in having help in using standardized outcome measures for documenting clients' progress?" Here there were only 5% of therapists and 3% of directors who were "not at all" interested. Of the therapists who never used outcome measures there were only 4% who had no interest in help. The overwhelming majority wanted help in multiple areas. The specific areas where you requested help are outlined in Table 2.4.

Table 2.4:   Areas of Requested Assistance in the Use of Standardized Outcome Measures

	Staff		Directors	
	Number	**%**	**Number**	**%**
Number of areas where help was requested				
None	7	5	2	3
Single area	17	12	6	9
Multiple areas	119	83	58	88
Specific areas where help was requested*				
List and characteristics of measures	121	85	60	91
Standardized forms and directions	105	73	49	74
Choosing measures	66	46	31	47
Communicating with other institutions doing similar things	59	41	34	52
Evaluating outcome in groups of clients	53	37	27	40
Evaluating outcome for multiprofessional programs	51	36	28	42
Setting up system	49	34	27	41

* Multiple responses permitted

The data were also reviewed to determine whether there were differences in your responses based on whether or not you used outcomes measures.

Of the 58 therapists using outcome measures, 81% were full-time, whereas only 62% of those not using outcome measures (n=38) were full-time. Directors were not asked if they were full-time or part-time. Only a very small proportion (7%) of therapists using outcome measures had only a diploma in physiotherapy, whereas 29% of those not using measures held only a diploma. The data indicated that therapists who use standardized outcome measures were more likely to hold a bachelor's degree, to be senior therapists, to have graduated after 1980, and to work in a department with more than 12 therapists. The characteristics of the directors whose departments use or do not use standardized outcome measures is less straightforward to describe as their characteristics relate more strongly to their status as directors and not necessarily to the use of outcome measures by the therapists in their departments.

Comparing users versus non-users of outcome measures, in regard to **areas of requested assistance** in their use, revealed more similarities than dissimilarities.

SOME DISCUSSION

The survey identified that **current practice involved only a limited use of outcome measures**. That is, even though 50% of therapists reported using these measures, a small proportion did not name any instruments and about 20% identified only one instrument and, even then, the psychometric properties of these instruments were underdeveloped. There was still evident confusion about what the term "published" meant. For many clinicians, the existence of a manual was sufficient for the scale to be considered as "published". For others, if their hospital bound and labelled a scale, this was also considered "published". In Table 2.5 the most frequently identified scales are listed.

Because the survey identified that **the major barrier** to use was lack of knowledge of available instruments and their properties, we are providing a description of the major instruments available to measure outcomes commonly used by physical therapists (these are described in Part III). Providing information on existing measures and their properties should reduce this barrier and, thus, achieve our objective of increasing the use of standardized outcome measures.

Table 2.5:   The Dominant Dozen

	Percent of therapists reporting use (n=143)
Manual Muscle Test	27
Berg Balance Scale	17
Visual Analogue Scale	16
Fugl-Meyer Assessment of Sensorimotor Recovery after Stroke	12
Functional Independence Measurement (FIM)	8
Range of Motion Measurement by Goniometer	8
Chedoke-McMaster Stroke Assessment	6
McGill Pain Questionnaire	5
Barthel Index of ADL	4
Motor Assessment Scale (for stroke)	3
Rancho Los Amigos Levels of Cognitive Function	2
Clinical Outcome Variable System (COVS)	2

Only a **small proportion of respondents were completely satisfied** with their current method of documenting clients' progress: 8% of therapists and 12% of directors. Some of these satisfied respondents were already using standardized outcome measures. Thus, of the whole sample of 209 therapists and directors, there is a resistant 7% who are still completely satisfied with documenting clients' progress without the use of standardized outcome measures.

One of the points you made clear in this survey is that though you want help, you **do not want a system of measurement imposed**. Instead, you wish to be able to choose those instruments that best meet your, and your clients', needs.

IN SUMMARY

Let's highlight once again what we found:

1. Current practice involves only a limited use of outcome measures.

2. Though 50% of therapists reported using these measures, a small proportion did not name any instruments and about 20% identified only one instrument.

3. Even then, the psychometric properties of these instruments were underdeveloped.

4. Two factors were associated with the use of standardized measures – holding a degree in physical therapy as opposed to a diploma, and working in a department with more than 12 therapists.

5. One of the major barriers to use was a lack of knowledge of available instruments and their properties.

6. Information provided on existing measures and their properties, therefore, should be able to reduce this barrier and, thus, we should have a stronger chance of encouraging therapists to increase their use of standardized outcome measures.

7. Only a small proportion of respondents were completely satisfied with their current method of documenting client's progress: 8% of therapists and 12% of directors.

8. They should be receptive to incorporating into their clinical practice the material developed in this book.

9. Emphatically therapists do not want a system of measurement imposed on them. Therapists want to be able to choose those instruments that best meet their measurement needs and the needs of their clients.

Surely now you will read and take seriously every word that follows!

PART III

The Heart of the Matter

In Part II you identified that one of the major barriers to the use of outcome measures was a lack of knowledge of available measures and their properties. This, the largest part of this book, is offered to help. It is presented as a guide and companion for all who aspire to improve their outcomes in physical therapy. It is neither the final word nor the bottom line. Only time and usage will reveal its practical value.

In the "Heart of the Matter" we do a number of things. First, we talk about the selection of outcome measures. Next, we present additional standards that, as users of measures, we hope you will follow. Then, to help enhance your ability to choose and review for yourself the instrument that best meets your needs and those of your clients, we provide a blank template for use when you do the reviewing. Next, for those of you who need a little support in this area, we've defined all the terminology so you can fill in the blanks yourself. Finally, we've reviewed measures in four specialty areas. The remainder of this part of the book – the Heart of the Matter – contains the review of the measures in four specialty areas – (A) Adult Neurological and Functional Activity, (B) Back and/or Pain, (C) Cardiopulmonary, (D) Developmental Paediatrics.

We chose these areas in the hope that there would be at least one measure of interest to each and every one of you. The individual expositions on the measures are laid out in coloured 2-page spreads to permit you to locate information easily. These 2-page spreads were carefully assembled and agonized over by our consultants and editors. The references are conveniently gathered at the book's end. Alas, we suspect that we have missed some important measures and not all the boxes contain positive and comforting data. Time will change that, but we have provided here, in the areas described above, the state-of-the-art and science of outcome measures in the first half of the 1990s.

Even if you are not an expert in statistics, you should be able to profit from a careful reading of these reviews, particularly in those fields that involve you most in clinical practice. Increasingly you will find the statistics make sense. Enjoy!

SELECTION OF OUTCOME MEASURES

"The validity of health status measures for the purpose of outcomes management is of vital interest to all professions engaged in medical rehabilitation, as well as to clients and the public."[1] The current lack of suitable validated measures for evaluating outcomes is a major problem – one that can only be addressed over time by the development and validation of new measures. In the meantime, clinicians should be aware of the measures in existence and of the relative properties of these measures. Whenever possible, the best of these standardized measures should be used on a regular basis and results made available across programs and centres.

STANDARDS FOR TESTS AND MEASURES

Standards for the use of measures by physical therapists currently exist. Four years of intensive effort by the American Physical Therapy Association's Task Force on "Standards for Tests and Measurements in Physical Therapy Practice" produced a landmark publication in 1991.[2] More recently the Advisory Group on Measurement Standards of the American Congress of Rehabilitation Medicine published a Supplement to the Archives of Physical Medicine and Rehabilitation on "Measurement Standards for Interdisciplinary Medical Rehabilitation".[1] That 23-page report not only speaks for itself, but fits with the objectives of this book so well that we have relied heavily upon it in this section. We also sought and received gracious permission from the editor to reprint for you the **General Standards for the Use of Measures**. They are described on pages 32 and 33 of this chapter. We would encourage those who feel ready to review them now. If you find some of the terminology difficult or aren't ready to jump in, read on and look at them after you've completed this chapter.

To aid users in the application of these standards, we developed the *Template* on pages 24-25 which is used throughout Part III of this book. A blank version of the template is provided for your use in the review of additional measures. To help with the complex task of mastering the application of the **General Standards for the Use of Measures,** we offer the following expansion on the terms used within the *Template*.

DESCRIPTION

Physical rehabilitation measures, like other health status instruments, can be thought of as having one (or more) of three purposes — *discriminative, predictive,* or *evaluative.*[3] The first of these purposes, *discrimination,* attempts to differentiate between people who, for example, do or do not have a particular trait or diagnosis. The second purpose, *prediction,* attempts to classify individuals into a set of predefined measurement categories for the purpose of estimating prognosis. This can be useful in treatment planning. The third purpose, *evaluation,* pertains to the measurement of change in an individual or group over time. This third purpose is the most relevant to outcome measurement.[4]

When reviewing a measure, summarize the content and indicate the purpose for which it is designed and validated, whether it is designed for clinical practice, for research, or both and whether it evaluates impairment, disability, and/or handicap.

Population

Generally, measures are developed and validated for use on a specific population, i.e. group of clients. This population should be described in sufficient detail that you can determine similarities and differences between the study's sample of clients and yours. Descriptions typically include age, diagnosis, setting, severity, and stage of the condition.

Time to Complete

Indicate the time required to administer, score, and interpret the test. Consider the practicality of the time for your setting.

Cost

Include the cost of purchasing the manual and any testing equipment that may be required. Consider whether the scoresheets are copyrighted or can be readily copied.

Training

Consider whether you have the necessary experience and/or professional qualifications to use the measure, and whether you can reliably apply it in your setting. If training beyond a basic level of familiarization with the measure is required (such as attendance at a course or seminar), indicate if this training is regionally available at a reasonable cost. Training guidelines should be specified in the test manual.

MEASURE _____

DESCRIPTION

Population	Time to Complete	Cost	Training

INSTRUCTIONS

SCALING

Format

Subscales

Scoring

RELIABILITY

Internal consistency

Test-retest Reliability

Interrater/Intrarater Reliability

VALIDITY

Content (domain or face)

Construct

Criterion

Predictive

Responsiveness

INSTRUCTIONS

Administration, scoring and score interpretation procedures should be given in either a test manual or other documentation. Assess the quality of the instructions given. Instructions should include information on required materials, test environment, directions on administering each item, and criteria for scoring and interpretation of total scores and subscores. Consider any potential harm, psychological or physical, that could result to a client, and consider whether the benefits outweigh the risks and costs.

SCALING

Format

Describe the administration format, paying particular attention to whether the measure has been designed and tested for use in the format that you need for your particular setting. Common formats include: *task performance or observation* – the client performs specific tasks while being observed by the one who administers the test, *self report* – the client is asked to report on their usual ability to carry out specific activities, *proxy or caregiver report* – report is given by another (e.g. parent, partner, or health-care worker) when the client cannot report for him or herself. For self or proxy report, indicate the *mode of report* – whether a verbal report is given as a face-to-face or a telephone interview, or whether a written response could be supplied as in a mailed questionnaire.

Subscales

Some measures have both an overall total score and subscores from various sections. Describe the individual test items and the content of each subscale. Indicate the number of items and summary score for each subscale.

Scoring

Individual items in most measures deal with either **attributes** (client characteristics) or with **behaviours** (activities). Examples of attributes are range of motion or muscle strength, and of behaviours are rolling over, sitting, or walking. Many methods exist for translating the attributes or behaviours, the items in the measure, into numbers. Item scores are combined, usually simply summed, into an overall score.[5] Commentary on scoring should indicate both the data type and how a total score is obtained.

How items in a measure are combined to determine an overall score depends on the *data type* used. This business of data type comes up again when you go to make a judgement about the appropriateness of the statistics used in the reliability and validation studies, so a brief description may be helpful to you.

There are four data types – *nominal, ordinal, interval,* or *ratio.*

Nominal, is simply a classification, for example, sex, race, or religion.

Ordinal data consists of ranked categories. A common example is to assign scores of 1 to 3 for mild, moderate and severe. The numbers assigned reflect the ordering of the categories, not the absolute value of each category. Purists suggest that ordinal scales cannot be aggregated to calculate overall scores, although this frequently is done. Everyone should be aware that though resulting errors may seem small, they may lead to incorrect conclusions.

In both *interval* and *ratio* scales (the difference between these two is that in the interval scale there is no meaningful zero such as in temperature), numbers reflect absolute values and these numbers can be added. In *ratio* scales which include a zero point, it is possible to multiply and divide scores; to state for example, that one score is twice another.[5] Most commonly, nominal data is not summed while interval, ordinal and ratio data are.

RELIABILITY

Reliability refers to a measure's repeatability when administered on more than one occasion or by more than one rater. As the "Standards" point out, users of measures should understand the types of reliability and how these qualities relate to clinical decisions.

Reliability also maybe defined as "the degree to which a measure is free from random error. The reliability of a measure is usually quantified in terms of the degree to which it renders consistent or reproducible results when properly administered under similar circumstances."[1] "Reliability should not be seen as a property which a particular instrument does or does not possess; rather any measure will have a certain degree of reliability when applied to certain populations under certain conditions. The issue which must be addressed for each type of reliability is how much is good enough."[6] Guidelines for how much reliability is "good enough" are suggested to range from correlations of 0.65[7] to 0.94.[4]

Types of reliability

There are several types of reliability which can be evaluated. These include *internal consistency, interrater, intrarater, and test-retest.* The selection depends on the purpose of the measure and the type of random error that one wants estimated.

Internal consistency refers to the way individual items of the instrument group together to form a unit. Consistent total scores are more likely with high internal consistency even if there is measurement error in one (or more) of the items. One way this property is evaluated is by examining how different halves of the instrument correlate (e.g. the correlation between odd and even numbered items).

Test-retest reliability, "or stability over time, is an important aspect of reliability, particularly with outcome measures."[1] The degree to which the scores change on repeated administration in the so called "stable" state should be taken into account when assessing "true" change over time.

Interrater reliability is the degree to which scores on a measure obtained by one trained observer agree with scores obtained by another trained observer. If trained individuals cannot agree, the assessment procedure is of doubtful use.[1]

Intrarater reliability is the degree to which scores on a measure obtained by one trained observer agree with the scores obtained when the same observer reapplies the measure at another time. This can be achieved either through test-retest or by videotaping the assessment and rescoring from the videotape.

Reliability Statistics

The statistic to be used to describe reliability depends upon the type of reliability and the data type – *nominal, ordinal, interval or ratio.*

Cronbach's coefficient alpha can be used to assess internal consistency.

Crude agreement is used with *nominal or ordinal* categories of responses. It is simply described in terms of percentage agreement.[1]

Kappa (K) should be used in assessments yielding multiple nominal categories, because it corrects for chance.[1]

Weighted K or *intra-class correlation coefficient (ICC)* are usually used to determine the reliability of a test when ratings are on an *ordinal* scale. Some authors suggest that with all quantitative scales – ordinal, interval or ratio, an analysis of variance (ANOVA) model and estimates of *intra-class correlation coefficients (ICC)* are possible and desirable.[8]

VALIDITY

Validity is the most important consideration when selecting a measure. Validity is commonly regarded as the extent to which a test measures what it is intended to measure. The term refers to the appropriateness, meaningfulness, and usefulness of a measure and of the inferences that can be made from the scores. A measure is validated by accumulating evidence that supports logical inferences made from the measure.[1]

Types of validity

The most common types of validity reported are *content, construct* and *criterion.*

Content validity is concerned with the extent to which items in a measure represent an adequate sampling of the content. [1]

Construct validity is the degree to which the scores obtained concur with the underlying theories related to the content – the theoretical constructs.[1] Constructs are concepts with multiple attributes and are embedded in theory. Establishing adequate construct validity requires piecing together a network of relationships. Specifically, construct validity is tested by (1) seeing whether a measure displays the pattern of converging or predictive relationships it should (convergent validity); (2) distinguishing the construct from confounding factors (divergent or discriminant validity); and (3) measuring with variations in settings, populations, and even details in measurement procedure so that generalization can be made beyond a narrow application.[1]

Criterion validity concerns the extent to which a measure is related to a "gold standard" or other external measures in the same domain. The two main types of this validity, *concurrent* and *predictive,* differ from the perspective of time.

Concurrent criterion validity is the degree to which a measure correlates with some important event or criterion occurring at the same time.

Predictive criterion validity is the extent to which a measure is able to forecast or predict an important future event or criterion.

Responsiveness

When the specific purpose of a measure is to evaluate outcome, a new type of validity – *responsiveness* – is emerging in the measurement literature. It deals with the notion of providing evidence of the ability of the measure to assess and quantify *clinically important change.*

Kirshner and Guyatt[3] first introduced this concept. More recent publications[4,9] suggest consideration of the following unique properties of evaluative measures:

- individual test items should be responsive to clinically important change
- the scale applied should have sufficient gradations to register change
- the measure should assess longitudinal change
- variations between replicate assessments should be small

- a strong relationship in change scores between a measure itself and external measures should exist

- the measure should be able to detect and quantify a clinically important difference

- instructions on interpretation of change scores should be adequately documented

Very few of the measures in this book have been developed specifically for use as evaluative measures, but over time we can expect to see much more validation specific to this use. More importantly, only a small number of measures now meet the standards that are currently being set. For the present, we can only select the best of those measures that are available, identify priority areas, and support the push for ongoing measurement development.

GENERAL STANDARDS FOR USE OF MEASURES*

- Users of measures should read the technical manual or relevant available documentation for measures they use and be familiar with relevant administration, scoring, and interpretation procedures, including reliability and validity for the specific application.

- Users of measures should understand the validity basis (content, criterion-oriented, and/or construct validity) for measures they use and select appropriate measures for specific applications accordingly.

- Users of measures should accurately portray the relevance of measures they use to the clinical assessment and decision-making process.

- Measures should be used by individuals who have the necessary training, experience, and/or professional qualifications.

- Training guidelines for examiners specified in the technical manual should be adhered to.

- Users of measures should know the population(s) for whom the measure was designed and should be able to logically justify the application of the measure to the population(s) they are assessing.

- Users of measures should know the population(s) and conditions from which normative data were collected to judge whether these data are applicable to the clients they are testing.

Reproduced with permission from the Archives of Physical Medicine & Rehabilitation.[1]

- Users of measures must consider potential harm, psychological or physical, that could result to a client from utilizing a measure. Users should determine whether the potential benefits to the client outweigh the risks before proceeding with the measurement.

- Users of measures should know the environmental conditions, equipment requirements, and procedures for correct administration and scoring of measures they choose and the effects upon results if these are altered. Users who deviate from the standardized accepted, or validated alternative protocols for administration or scoring of measure should not use published data or documentation of reliability, validity, or normal values for interpretation of results unless the user can provide evidence that the procedural deviations do not compromise reliability or validity.

- Users of measures should consider the sensitivity, specificity, pretest probability, and prognostic validity of tests that categorize or diagnose the person tested.

- When tests that do not meet measurement standards are used, users should express appropriate cautions and reservations when interpreting test results.

- Users of measures should understand types of reliability and validity and how these qualities relate to clinical decisions and other use of measurements.

- When selecting measures, users should consider their practicality in terms of personnel, time, equipment, space, cost and impact on the client.

THE MEASURES

Table of Outcome Measures

A. Adult Motor and Functional Activity Measures

A1. Timed "Up and Go"
2. Modified Sphygmomanometer for Measuring Muscle Strength ("Modified Sphyg")
3. Activity Index
4. Motor Assessment Scale (MAS)
5. Chedoke-McMaster Stroke Assessment (Chedoke)
6. Action Research Arm Test
7. Berg Balance Scale
8. The Barthel Index
9. Functional Independence Measure (FIM)
10. The Fugl-Meyer Assessment of Sensorimotor Recovery After Stroke
11. Katz Index of Activities of Daily Living
12. Kenny Self-Care Evaluation
13. Klein-Bell Activities of Daily Living Scale
14. Level of Rehabilitation Scale (LORS-II)
15. The PULSES Profile
16. Rivermead Motor Assessment (RMA)
17. Rivermead ADL Assessment
18. The Functional Autonomy Measurement System (SMAF)
19. Patient Evaluation Conference System (PECS)
20. The Canadian Neurological Scale (CNS)
21. Clinical Outcome Variable Scale (COVS)

(Also refer to Measures B4, B5; C8, C9.)

B. Back and/or Pain Measures

B1. Visual Analogue Scale (VAS)
2. Numeric Pain Rating Scale (NPRS)
3. Pain Drawing
4. Sickness Impact Profile (SIP)
5. Disability Questionnaire (DQ)
6. Oswestry Low Back Pain Disability Questionnaire
7. Partial Sit-up/Curl-up as a Test of Abdominal Muscle Strength/Endurance
8. Sorensen Test for Endurance of the Back Musculature
9. Pressure Biofeedback (PBF) for Measuring Muscular Endurance of the Transverse Abdominal and Abdominal Oblique Musculature
10. Modified Schober Method of Measuring Spinal Mobility
11. Leighton Flexometer for Measuring Spinal Mobility
12. Inclinometer Method of Measuring Spinal Mobility
13. Lifting Dynamometers
14. Isokinetic Dynamometers

(Also refer to Measures A2 and C9.)

C. Cardiopulmonary Measures

C1. Heart Rate
2. Blood Pressure
3. Respiratory Rate
4. Percussion
5. Auscultation of Lung Sounds
6. Chronic Respiratory Disease Questionnaire
7. Visual Analogue Scale for Dyspnea
8. Six-Minute Walking Test
9. Self-Paced Walking Test to Predict VO_2 max
10. Vital Capacity
11. Peak Expiratory Flow Rate (PEFR)
12. Maximum Inspiratory and Expiratory Pressures (MIP's/MEP's or MIF/MEF or PImax/PEmax)
13. Oxygen Saturation

D. Developmental Measures

D1. Alberta Infant Motor Scale (AIMS)
2. Bayley Scales of Infant Development (Psychomotor Scale)
3. Peabody Developmental Motor Scales
4. Test of Motor and Neurological Functions (TMNF)
5. Test of Motor Impairment
6. Posture and Fine Motor Assessment of Infants (PFMAI)
7. Basic Gross Motor Assessment (BGMA)
8. Bruininks-Oseretsky Test of Motor Proficiency (BOTMP)
9. Gross Motor Function Measure (GMFM)
10. Gross Motor Performance Measure (GMPM)
11. Movement Assessment of Infants (MAI)
1 2. Pediatric Evaluation of Disability Inventory (PEDI)

A.1.   Timed "Up and Go"

DESCRIPTION

The Timed Up and Go test is a quick and practical method of testing basic mobility manoeuvres. It can be used both clinically and for research purposes.[1]

Population	Time to Complete	Cost	Training
The frail elderly, with a wide variety of physical conditions: stroke, Parkinson's disease, rheumatoid arthritis, osteoarthritis, multiple sclerosis, hip fracture, cerebellar degeneration, and general deconditioning.	A few minutes.	None, except that a stop watch is required.	None required.

INSTRUCTIONS

Simple directions are provided.

SCALING

Format

Task performance.

Subscales

The tests consists of one multiphase task. The client begins seated in a chair. He/she is asked to rise from an arm chair, stand still momentarily, walk to a line on the floor 3 meters away, turn, return, turn around and sit down again.

Scoring

The client is scored according to the time in seconds required to complete the task. The observer's perception of the client's risk of falling is rated on a 5-point ordinal scale.

1. Normal
2. Very slightly abnormal
3. Mildly abnormal
4. Moderately abnormal
5. Severely abnormal

RELIABILITY

Internal consistency

N/A

Test-retest Reliability

Twenty geriatric clients were evaluated by the same observer on consecutive visits and the agreement was extremely high (ICC 0.99).[1]

Interrater Reliability

Twenty-two geriatric clients were evaluated separately by 3 raters on the same day and the agreement on the time to complete the task was very high (ICC 0.99).[2] Forty clients aged 52-94 years of age were tested and videotaped by the physiotherapists and doctors. The agreement on time was high for the physiotherapists and moderate for the physicians (Kendall's coefficient W, 0.85 and 0.69, respectively).[1]

VALIDITY

Content (domain or face)

Not reported.

Construct

Not reported.

Concurrent

Forty clients were tested on the Up and Go test, a laboratory measure of balance (sway path) and gait speed. Correlations with the sway path were poor (0.5) and with gait speed moderate (0.75).[1] Twenty-two clients were also tested on the Up and Go test, and several other measures of balance and function. A curvilinear relationship was found between the Up and Go test and the Berg Balance Scale (-0.72), gait speed (-0.55) and the Barthel Index (-0.51).[1] The correlations were predictably negative indicating that the longer the time for the Up and Go test, the lower was the score on the Berg Balance Scale, the Barthel Index and gait speed.

Predictive

Not reported.

Responsiveness

Not reported.

IMPORTANT REFERENCES ARE FOUND ON PAGE 181.

A.2. Modified Sphygmomanometer for Measuring Muscle Strength ("Modified Sphyg")

DESCRIPTION

The instrument devised by Helewa, Goldsmith, and Smythe[1,2] is a modified aneroid sphygmomanometer in which the bladder has been removed from the cuff. The bladder is folded into 3 sections and placed in a cotton bag. Testing is done isometrically, in similar body positions to those used in manual muscle testing. The modified sphyg has been used as a clinical outcome measure. It has been used to test a number of different muscle groups including the abdominal musculature.

Population	Time to Complete	Cost	Training
Rheumatoid arthritis population and back injured individuals.	Less than 2 min.	Approximately $50.	Practice time to ensure good technique and reproducibility.

INSTRUCTIONS

The subject must be able to perform a resisted isometric contraction. A baseline pressure is set on the "modified sphyg". The bag is held between the tester's hand and the body part. A resisted isometric contraction is performed by the individual and the force is matched by the tester. The test is performed 3 times. Suggested protocols are provided in the literature (Helewa et al).[1,2] They require practice for good results.

SCALING

Format

Task performance.

Subscales

None.

Scoring

The maximum pressure reached, in mmHg, is recorded. The test is performed 3 times and the mean is calculated.

RELIABILITY

Internal consistency

N/A

Test-retest Reliability

Not reported.

Interrater Reliability

An analysis of variance showed no statistically significant difference between raters (p > 0.05).[1]

VALIDITY

Content (domain or face)

The test only accounts for static strength in the range tested and doesn't account for dynamic strength.

Construct

Construct validity is good. Muscle strength is the measure of the force generated by a muscle. The "modified sphyg" measures the amount of pressure exerted at one point in range.

Concurrent

Concurrent validity is high. A correlation of 0.94 (p < 0.02) was found between the "modified sphyg" and free weights used to determine a 1 repetition maximum.[1]

Predictive

Not reported.

Responsiveness

Although one study found the relative sensitivity did not reach statistically significant levels,[1] other authors have found the "modified sphyg" to be a sensitive measurement tool. In a single case study, it was sensitive to the expected changes due to treatment.[3] The mean values were significantly different between a group of normal individuals and a group of individuals with low back pain.[2] The "modified sphyg" was found to have a sensitivity of 5% and a specificity of 5%.[2]

IMPORTANT REFERENCES ARE FOUND ON PAGE 181.

A.3. Activity Index

DESCRIPTION

The Activity Index was developed to measure the effectiveness of an activity program for stroke clients. It measures mental capacity as well as motor activity and ADL function.[1] The Activity Index is intended to be used to develop treatment strategies and to measure change in functional capacity during the first year following stroke.

Population	Time to Complete	Cost	Training
Stroke clients, adult population.	Up to 1 hour.	No special materials.	None required.

INSTRUCTIONS

A list of items is presented but no information regarding the criteria for scoring the items is given.

SCALING

Format

Task Performance, or client or caregiver report.

Subscales

The Activity Index is divided into 3 subscales:
1. Mental Capacity (32 points)
2. Motor activity measured from a functional point of view (24 points)
3. ADL function ambulation, hygiene, dressing, feeding, continence (36 points)

Scoring

The response for each item is given a score ranging from 1 to 12 points for a maximum of 92 points. The scoring system is not the same for all items. Higher values imply a higher level of function.

RELIABILITY

Internal consistency (split halves)

For the most part, the tests of homogeneity (Cronbach alpha) indicated an acceptable degree of internal consistency as indicated below.

Total test	0.94
Mental subscale	0.83
Motor subscale	0.79
ADL subscale	0.94

In addition the correlations between the motor and ADL subscales were high (0.85); however, the correlations between the mental scale and the other two subscales were lower: mental and motor 0.64, mental and ADL 0.76.

Test-retest Reliability

Not reported.

Interrater Reliability

Not reported.

VALIDITY

Content (domain or face)

Not reported.

Construct

Factor analysis was performed. 68.7% of the variance of the variables could be explained by two factors: factor 1 represented motor activity of the right extremity and factor 2 represented motor activity of the left extremity.

Concurrent

One hundred and twelve clients were evaluated 48 hours post-stroke on both the Activity Index and the Rankin Disability Scale. The correlation between these 2 scales was high (0.94).[1]

Predictive

The Activity Index scores at 48 hours post-stroke were examined according to later outcome:

0 - Dead	2 - Medium score 50-83
1 - Low score <50	3 - High score >83

Linear regression was used to measure the predictive ability of the Activity Index $r^2 = 3 - 44\%$ for clients in the experimental group (more intensive activation program during the first 4 weeks) and 45-61% for the control group (p.<001). Better relationship was found at 3 weeks and at discharge as compared to follow up measures.

IMPORTANT REFERENCES ARE FOUND ON PAGE 181.

A.4. Motor Assessment Scale (MAS)

DESCRIPTION

The Motor Assessment Scale was designed to measure the motor recovery of clients following stroke using relevant and functional motor activities. It quantifies the motor progress of stroke clients, using a quick and easy administered evaluation. The MAS was designed for clinical practice and for research.[1]

Population	Time to Complete	Cost	Training
Stroke clients, adult population.	15-30 minutes.	Minimal - a few common items are required.	None required.

INSTRUCTIONS
A general description of the administration of the scale is provided. The criteria for scoring each point for every item are described in detail.

SCALING

Format

Task performance.

Subscales

The assessment evaluates eight areas of motor function and one test of muscle tone:

Motor function   supine side lying
supine to sitting over side of bed
balance sitting
sitting to standing
walking
upper arm function
hand movements
advanced hand activities

Muscle tone

Timing of some items is included in order to assess quality of performance.

Scoring

Scoring is based on a 7-point ordinal scale for a maximum score of 48.

Motor function   0 - unable to perform
1 - optimal motor behaviour

Muscle tone   >4 - hypertonus
<4 - hypotonus
4 - normal

Each item is rated 3 times and the best response is used.

RELIABILITY

Internal consistency

Not reported.

Test-retest Reliability

Fourteen stroke clients aged 42-85 years were evaluated twice within 4 weeks. Correlations between the results were high (0.72-0.97).[1]

Interrater Reliability

Physical therapists and students rated videotapes of evaluations on the Motor Assessment Scale 6 to 40 weeks post-stroke. The resultant scores were compared to one Gold Standard Scoring. High correlations were found (0.89-0.99).[1]

Two evaluators rated 24 evaluations with excellent correlations found on the motor function test (0.95-0.99). Correlations for the tone subsection was poor (0.29).[2]

VALIDITY

Content (domain or face)

Not reported.

Construct

Not reported.

Concurrent

The Motor Assessment Scale for stroke and the Fugl-Meyer Assessment for stroke were administered to 30 clients 6 to 96 months post-stroke on consecutive days. Separate examiners were used for each evaluation. Correlation for the total score was high (0.88), but extremely variable for the individual items (0.28-0.82).[2]

Predictive

Fifty acute stroke clients were tested on a modified version of the MAS. The one-week post-stroke scores from balance sitting, the arm, age and bowel control explained 85% of the variance in outcome in the Barthel Index of ADL at one month post-stroke.[3,4]

Responsiveness

Not reported.

IMPORTANT REFERENCES ARE FOUND ON PAGE 181.

A.5. Chedoke-McMaster Stroke Assessment (Chedoke)

DESCRIPTION

The Chedoke-McMaster Stroke Assessment (Chedoke) was developed to determine the presence and severity of physical impairment following stroke, to classify clients for treatment and research purposes, to predict rehabilitation outcomes and to measure clinically important change in physical disability.[1] It includes both a physical impairment inventory and a disability inventory. Its scoring is based on classifying recovery post-stroke using an expansion and modification of the stages described by Brunnstrom. The Chedoke was designed to be used in conjunction with the Uniform Data System for Medical Rehabilitation (UDS).

Population	Time to Complete	Cost	Training
Adult stroke clients.	Approximately 1 hour.	Test manual $50.	None required.

INSTRUCTIONS

The detailed test manual provides instructions for administering and scoring. The manual describes the development and validation work to date and, as well, gives suggestions for therapeutic activities.

SCALING

Format

Task performance.

Subscales

The assessment consists of (1) an impairment inventory with 6 subscales: the stage of recovery of postural control, the arm, hand, leg, foot and shoulder pain. (2) a disability inventory with 2 subscales: (gross motor function 10 items evaluating rolling, sitting, transferring and standing) and walking (5 items).

Scoring

Scoring of the physical impairment inventory is based on a 7-point ordinal scale corresponding to the 7 stages of motor recovery. For each stage of motor recovery beyond stage 1, 3 activities are given. If the person is able to achieve 2 of these 3 activities, they are considered to be in this stage of recovery. The physical impairment inventory, having 6 dimensions, has a maximum total score of 42 and a minimum score of 6. The disability index has a maximum score of 100: 7 points for each of the first 14 items, and 2 points for item 15 (2-minute walk test). Minimum score is 14. Eight points change on the disability inventory equates to clinically important change as judged by client and caregiver.

RELIABILITY

Internal consistency – Not reported.

Test-retest Reliability – Clients were assessed on the disability inventory upon admission and again within five days. ICCs ranged from 0.96 - 0.98 for the subscales and total score was 0.98.[1]

Intrarater Reliability – The physical impairment assessments of 32 stroke clients, (mean age of 64) were videotaped during the first week of admission. The treating therapist scored the admission evaluation and then the videotape after a minimum interval of 2 weeks. ICCs for 6 dimensions were 0.93-0.98 total score was 0.98.[1]

Interrater Reliability – The 32 clients were scored on the physical impairment scale and the disability inventory by two physical therapists during week 1 of admission. The physical impairment inventory ICCs were 0.85 - 0.96 and total score 0.97. ICCs for disability index were 0.98 for individual items and 0.99 for total score.[1]

VALIDITY

Content (domain or face) Not reported.

Construct – Construct validity assessed for the 32 clients. Specific items on the impairment and disability inventories were compared with similar attributes on other measures: impairment with Fugl-Meyer, and disability with FIM. The correlations were:

Chedoke	Fugl-Meyer	r	p
shoulder	upper limb pain	0.76	<0.01
postural control	balance	0.84	<0.01
leg and foot	balance	0.84	<0.001
arm and hand	shoulder, elbow, forearm wrist and hand	0.95	<0.001

Chedoke's gross motor function correlated with mobility on the FIM (r = 0.90, p <0.001); walking index correlated with locomotion (r = 0.85, p < .01).[1]

Concurrent – The same 32 clients were evaluated on admission and discharge on the Chedoke and the Fugl-Meyer and FIM scales. The impairment inventory of the Chedoke correlated highly with the Fugl-Meyer (r = 0.95, p < .001), however, the disability inventory and the FIM only showed a moderate correlation (r = 0.79, p <0.05).[1,2]

Predictive – The gross motor function index is a strong predictor of living arrangement following discharge. Predictive equations suitable for use when planning treatment are available.

Responsiveness – The disability inventory was compared to the FIM on ability to detect clinically important change. The variance ratio (variance due to change/variance due to change + error)[1] for the results of the change between admission and discharge scores was 0.53 for the disability inventory and 0.39 for the FIM suggesting that the disability inventory is more responsive to change than the FIM. The relative efficiency was 1.92 times greater, hence a smaller sample size is needed to detect similar degrees of change with Chedoke.[1]

IMPORTANT REFERENCES ARE FOUND ON PAGE 182.

A.6.   Action Research Arm Test

DESCRIPTION

The Action Research Arm Test is a measure of the functional recovery of the upper limb in clients with hemiplegia due to cortical involvement. It is based on an assessment developed by Carroll.[1] Motor actions, including arm movements and hand functions, are assessed. The Action Research Arm Test can be used clinically and in research.

Population	Time to Complete	Cost	Training
Hemiplegic clients with upper limb involvement, specifically, those with CVA, cortical surgery and closed head injury.	About 8 minutes.	Minimal (several common objects required).	None required.

INSTRUCTIONS

A description of the materials required is provided, but specific directions for the administration of each of the test items are not included.

SCALING

Format

Task Performance.

Subscales

The test is divided into four domains. The items are arranged in order of difficulty:

Grasp - lift blocks, ball, stone from one shelf of trolley to another (6 items)
Grip - pour, displace tube, washer over bolt (4 items)
Pinch - ball and marble from one shelf to another (6 items)
Gross movement - hand behind head, hand on top of head, hand to
mouth (4 items)

Scoring

Items are scored on a 4-point ordinal scale for a maximum of 60 points.

0 - cannot perform any part of the test
1 - can partially perform test
2 - can complete test but took abnormally long or had great difficulty
3 - performs test normally

RELIABILITY

Internal consistency

Not reported.

Test-retest Reliability

Twenty clients, aged 26-72 years were tested twice with a mean interval of 7.5 days. Correlation between the two tests was high (0.98).[2]

Interrater Reliability

Twenty clients, with cortical damage were scored by one examiner and one rater. Correlation was high (0.99).[2]

VALIDITY

Content (domain or face)

Not reported.

Construct

The items follow a Guttman scale:

	Reproducibility	Scalability
Grasp	.98	.94
Grip	.99	.94
Pinch	.99	.94
Gross movement	.98	.97

Concurrent

Fifty-three clients aged 47 to 88 years, in the acute stages of stroke were tested on the Action Research Arm Test and the Fugl-Meyer. Correlations between the test scores were high at both 2 weeks (0.91) and 8 weeks (0.94) post-stroke.[3]

Predictive

Not reported.

Responsiveness

Not reported.

IMPORTANT REFERENCES ARE FOUND ON PAGE 182.

A.7. Berg Balance Scale

DESCRIPTION

The Berg Balance Scale[1-3] is an objective measure of balance abilities. The test has been used to identify and evaluate balance impairment in the elderly.

Population	Time to Complete	Cost	Training
The elderly client with stroke, Parkinson's disease and other causes of balance impairment.	15 - 20 min.	Nominal.	None required.

INSTRUCTIONS

The directions for items are provided on the scoring sheet.

SCALING

Format

Task Performance.

Subscales

The scale consists of 14 tasks common in everyday life. The items test the subject's ability to maintain positions or movements of increasing difficulty by diminishing the base of support from sitting, standing, to single leg stance. The ability to change positions is also assessed. Each item is scored on a scale from 0-4, for a minimum of 56 points.

Scoring

Scoring is based on a 5-point ordinal scale.

A score of 4 - performs movements independently and holds position for the prescribed time or performed within a set time frame. 0 – unable to perform item. A description of the criteria for scoring each level is provided.

RELIABILITY

Internal consistency

Fourteen clients aged 65 and over displaying varying degrees of balance impairment were videotaped while performing the 14 movements on the scale. Cronbach's alpha for the total score was 0.96. Individual items ranged from 0.72 - 0.90. Correlations ranged from 0.38 to 0.94.

Intrarater Reliability

Four therapists rated the same videotape again, one week later. The ICC for the total score was 0.99, ranging from 0.71 to 0.99 for the individual items.[2,3]

Interrater Reliability

Five physiotherapists and one test administrator rated the evaluations of the same 14 clients. The ICC for the total score was excellent (0.99), and was good to excellent for the individual items (0.71 - 0.99).[2,3]

VALIDITY

Content (domain or face)

The items were selected based on interview with 10 professionals and 12 geriatric clients. The list of items was revised following a pretest of all preliminary items.

Construct

Seventy acute stroke clients were tested on the Berg Balance Scale, the Barthel, and the Fugl-Meyer Scale at 4, 6 and 12 weeks post-stroke. Correlations between the Berg Scale and the Barthel were 0.80 - 0.94, and 0.62 - 0.94 for the Fugl-Meyer.[2,3]

Concurrent

The score of 23 clients on the Berg Balance Scale were correlated with the global ratings provided by caregivers (poor, fair, good). Spearman correlations were significant, with only 4 pairs of observation not corresponding.

Correlations between scores on the Berg Balance Scale and ratings of 113 residents of a home for the elderly and their caregivers ranged from poor to good (elderly: 0.39 to 0.41; caregivers 0.47 to 0.61).

Thirty one elderly clients were measured on the Berg Balance Scale, lab measures of postural sway and clinical measures of balance and mobility. Correlations for sway were -0.55, clinical measures -0.46 to -0.67, Tinetti balance subscale 0.91, Barthel mobility subscale 0.67, Up and Go Test -0.76.

Predictive

One hundred and thirteen elderly were followed for 12 months, and were classified as having 0, 1, = > 2 falls during that time. A Berg Balance Scale of < 45 was predictive of multiple falls.

Responsiveness

The Berg Balance Scale discriminated between subjects according to their use of mobility aids (walker, cane, none). It was also found to differentiate between outcomes for groups of stroke clients. At 12 weeks post-stroke, scores were highest for those at home, lowest for those still in hospital and intermediate for clients in rehabilitation centers.

IMPORTANT REFERENCES ARE FOUND ON PAGE 182.

A.8. The Barthel Index

DESCRIPTION

The index was developed to monitor functional independence before and after treatment, and to indicate the amount of nursing care needed.[1] It was intended for long-term clients, but has also been used as an evaluative measure. The Barthel can be used clinically, to monitor changes in function, and for research. The Barthel has been used on clients with stroke, spinal cord injuries, other neurological conditions, burns, cardiac problems and amputations.[2-20]

Population	Time to Complete	Cost	Training
Adult population, all diagnoses.	20 minutes if performance observed; 5 minutes if verbal information by client.	Minimal.	May be completed by any health care professional, or trained interviewer or even the client.

INSTRUCTIONS

Provided for scoring each of the levels of independence for each item.

SCALING

Format

Interview   Telephone Administration
Observation   Self Report
Medical Records

Subscales

Ten Activities are assessed:
Feeding   Ascend and descend stairs
Moving from wheelchair to bed and return   Dressing
Personal hygiene   Controlling bowels
Getting on and off toilet   Controlling bladder
Bathing self
Walking on level surface/propel wheelchair

Scoring

A score of 0, 5, 10 or 15 is assigned to each level, for a total of 100 points. The items are weighted differently. The scores reflect the amount of time and assistance a client requires. Granger et al[2-6] reported that 60 represents the cutoff between independence and more marked dependence. Forty or below indicates severe dependence and 20 or below reflects total dependence. The Granger Adapted Barthel consists of 15 items rated on a 4-point ordinal. Shah[16] modified the Barthel to increase its sensitivity to detect changes by increasing the number of categories used to record improvement.

RELIABILITY

Internal consistency

Not reported.

Interrater Reliability

The medical charts of severely disabled adults were reviewed. The correlation between reviews was high (0.89).

In the evaluation of stroke clients, correlations between raters was high (>.95) for the total score and moderate to high for the individual scores (0.71 - 1.00).[21]

The self rating by 30 rehabilitation clients differed significantly from assessments performed by therapists, with the clients rating themselves lower than the therapists.[12]

Twenty neurorehabilitation clients, aged 18-86 years were scored on the Barthel by a physician and an occupational therapist. Correlations between the test scores were high (.88 - .99).[20]

VALIDITY

Content (domain or face)

The evaluation tests most functions thought to comprise Activities of Daily Living.

Construct

Not reported.

Concurrent

Barthel admission scores correlate moderately with Barthel discharge scores (.75),[8] and for upper extremity function (0.64).

Predictive

Evaluation of spinal cord injured rehabilitation clients at admission, discharge and 12 months later resulted in a linear regression r^2 of .89.[15] When 84 stroke clients from 8 rehabilitation centers were tested on the Granger adapted Barthel, the scores were predictive of living arrangement status.[10]

The percentage of stroke clients who died within the first 6 months following admission decreased significantly as Barthel admission scores increased. They were predictive of length of stay and client's subsequent progress.[18]

Responsiveness

One thousand and twenty-five clients with a mean age of 64 years, were evaluated at admission and discharge. A higher percentage of clients with scores higher than 60 at admission improved over the time period as compared to those with initial scores less than 60 (77% versus 36%).[19]

IMPORTANT REFERENCES ARE FOUND ON PAGE 183.

A.9.   Functional Independence Measure (FIM)

DESCRIPTION

The FIM, an assessment instrument of functional status, is part of the Uniform Data Set for Medical Rehabilitation (UDS). It can be used clinically as an outcome measure.[1-5]

Population	Time to Complete	Cost	Training
All rehabilitation clients.	30 minutes.	Minimal.	Workshops to train users and test reliability are available.

INSTRUCTIONS
Extensive manual for U.D.S. for Medical Rehabilitation available: 82 Farber Hall, SUNY-South Campus, Buffalo, NY 14214

SCALING

Format

Task performance.

Subscales

The FIM consists of 23 items in 7 areas of function:
Self Care (6 items)
Sphincter control (2 items)
Mobility (3 items)
Locomotion (3 items)
Communication (2 items)
Social adjustment/cooperation (4 items)
Cognition/problem solving (3 items)

Scoring

The client is scored as:

7.	Independent	• complete
6.		• modified
5.	Dependent	• modified requires supervision
4.		• modified requires minimal assistance
3.		• modified requires moderate assistance
2.		• requires maximal assistance
1.		• complete

RELIABILITY

Internal consistency

Not reported.

Test-retest Reliability

Not reported.

Interrater Reliability

One hundred and twenty-seven newly injured spinal cord clients at 13 centres were assessed by 2 raters at admission and discharge. Correlations were high (0.83 - 0.96).

VALIDITY

Content (domain or face)

Eight different disciplines involving 114 clinicians evaluated 110 clients to ensure face validity.

Construct

Not reported.

Concurrent

Forty-one spinal cord injured clients were evaluated within 45 days post-injury, on the Modified Barthel and modified FIM (only Self care - feeding, grooming, bathing, dressing upper body, dressing lower body, perineal care, and Mobility - chair transfer, toilet transfer, tub transfer, walking, wheelchair propulsion). One nurse clinician tested the clients upon admission to rehabilitation, discharge from rehabilitation and at 12 month follow up.[4]

		Correlation
r^2	Self-care	.89 - .94
	Mobility	.64 - .76
	Total	.83 - .89

Predictive

The FIM was found to be the most useful tool in predicting burden of care as measured in minutes of assistance provided by another person to clients with multiple sclerosis. In addition, the FIM contributes to predicting the subjects's level of satisfaction with life.

Responsiveness

Scores on the FIM for 127 spinal cord injured clients changed from admission to discharge (41 - 52%). In a study of clients with multiple sclerosis, the FIM was found to be more sensitive in describing levels of disability and more precise in defining items than the Incapacity Status Scale.[1]

IMPORTANT REFERENCES ARE FOUND ON PAGE 184.

A.10. Fugl-Meyer Assessment of Sensorimotor Recovery After Stroke

DESCRIPTION

The Fugl-Meyer Assessment evaluates change in motor impairment following stroke.[1] It tests motor recovery, balance, sensation and joint range of motion. The test may be used for treatment planning, to evaluate the effectiveness of a rehabilitation program and for research. Evaluators need to be skilled in the evaluation of the quality of movement, and must be familiar with the test items.

Population	Time to Complete	Cost	Training
Stroke clients, adult population.	10-20 minutes.	Minimal. A few common items are required.	Evaluation skill required.

INSTRUCTIONS

Specific directions for the administration of each item, the client's position and the instructions provided to the clients, as well as the criteria for scoring are provided.

SCALING

Format

Task performance.

Subscales

The evaluation is divided into three subscales:
Motor Function
Upper extremity - shoulder/elbow/forearm/wrist/hand
Lower extremity - hip/knee/ankle, reflex activity
coordination/speed
Balance
Sensation
Passive Joint Motion/Joint Pain

Scoring

Scoring is on a 3-point ordinal scale for a maximum total score of 226.

0 - cannot perform
2 - performs fully

The specific requirements for scoring each of the items differs based on the type of item. The total scores for the subsections of the test do not all add up to the reported total in several publications.

RELIABILITY

Internal consistency

Not reported.

Test-retest Reliability

Nineteen stroke clients aged 34-76 years of age at least 1 year post-stroke were tested 3 times using the Fugl-Meyer assessment. Correlations between the test scores were excellent (total: 0.98 - 0.99; subtests 0.87 - 1.00). ANOVAS found no significant difference on either the total score or any of the subsections.[2]

Interrater Reliability

Eighteen stroke clients were tested on the upper extremity and lower extremity subsections of the test. ANOVAS found no significant differences between the raters' scores on the lower extremity and the upper extremity total scores, but the coordination and reflex scores did differ significantly.[2]

VALIDITY

Content (domain or face)

Not reported.

Construct

The Fugl-Meyer assessment is based on Twitchell's concept that after a stroke, motor recovery (if it occurs), follows a predictable sequence dependent on limb synergies. The Brunnstrom stages of recovery provided the basis for item selection in the motor subsection.

The internal validity of the test is supported by the finding that the order of sequential stages of motor return has been validated.[3]

Concurrent

The Fugl-Meyer and DeSouza methods were used to assess 50 clients with stroke resulting in an upper extremity deficit. Correlations between the two tests were excellent (0.95) (multiple regression analysis r = 0.97).[4] 15 male stroke clients aged 46-87 years, one month to 11 years post-stroke were evaluated on the Fugl-Meyer and Barthel assessments. Correlations were moderate (0.67 - 0.76).[5] Correlations with the Action Research Arm Test, from the evaluation of 53 acute stroke clients 47-88 years of age, were excellent (2 weeks – 0.91; 8 weeks – 0.94).

Predictive

Not reported.

Responsiveness

Not reported.

IMPORTANT REFERENCES ARE FOUND ON PAGE 185.

A.11. Katz Index of Activities of Daily Living

DESCRIPTION

This is a measure of function in activities of daily living used to objectively evaluate chronically ill and aging populations. It takes an interdisciplinary approach.[1] Although developed specifically for the elderly, especially with hip fractures, it has been used with a variety of chronic conditions: stroke, multiple sclerosis, arthritis, malignancy, amputations, cardiovascular disease, spinal cord injuries, peripheral neuropathy, cerebral palsy, Parkinson's disease. It has also been used with children and to evaluate severity of chronic illness and effectiveness of treatment.

Population	Time to Complete	Cost	Training
All adults, children.	Not reported.	Common everyday objects used.	Not reported.

INSTRUCTIONS

The definition of what is classified as independent as well as the specific requirements for scoring an item as independent is provided for each item on the ADL form.

SCALING

Format

Task performance (also can score on history of known performance) - Interview.

Subscales

Each discipline on the team records the results for their area of assessment on their own data sheet. All data sheets are sent to a central file where they are put together on one data sheet. The test consists of 6 subscales:

Bathing	Transferring
Dressing	Continence
Going to the toilet	Feeding

Scoring

Each category is rated as dependent or independent. The client's overall performance is then summarized on an 8-point ordinal scale. Clients are grouped according to independence in the 6 key personal areas.

Class A - Independent in all areas
Class B - Independent in all but 1 function
Class C - Independent in all but bathing and 1 additional function
Class D - Independent in all but bathing, dressing and 1 additional function
Class E - Independent in all but bathing, dressing, going to the toilet and 1 additional function
Class F - Independent in all but bathing, dressing, going to the toilet, transferring and 1 additional function
Class G - Dependent in all 6 functions
Other   - Dependent in 2 or more functions that do not fit into any other category

RELIABILITY

Internal consistency

Not reported.

Test-retest Reliability

Not reported.

Interrater Reliability

Four observers (nurses) rated 100 clients and reported high interrater reliability (values not reported).[2]

VALIDITY

Content (domain or face)

The order of recovery of function is in order of ascending complexity and is similar to the development of function in a child.

Construct

When 4 observers rated 100 clients the coefficient of scalability was moderate to high (0.74-0.76 and 0.81-0.88), suggesting the Katz Index forms a successful cumulative scale.[2]

Concurrent

Not reported.

Predictive

The Katz was used to evaluate 230 stroke clients, aged 31-96 years. It predicted who would be living at home at 1 month.[3]

Sensitivity - 83-94%
Specificity - 97%
Positive predictive power 94-96%
Negative predictive power 92-96%

One hundred and fifty-four stroke and hip fracture inpatients were tested post-injury, 79% of those clients who obtained a score of D,E,F, or G were non-family care; 45% of those with B or C in non-family care and 0% of A were in non-family care.[4]

Responsiveness

Not reported.

IMPORTANT REFERENCES ARE FOUND ON PAGE 186.

A.12. Kenny Self-Care Evaluation

DESCRIPTION

The Kenny was designed to measure the ability to function independently in ADL, specifically in self care skills, for setting goals and for rating client's progress over time in the home or other protected environment. It covers a narrower scope than most other ADL scales, but each topic is covered in detail.[1-3]

Population	Time to Complete	Cost	Training
Institutionalized and hospitalized adult clients.	Not indicated.	Not indicated.	None required.

INSTRUCTIONS

Not indicated.

SCALING

Format

Task performance.

Subscales

The 17 self care activities are divided into 7 categories with 85 component tasks:

Bed activities - moving in bed, rising and sitting
Transfers - sitting transfer, standing transfer, toilet transfer, bathing transfer
Locomotion - walking (with or without equipment), stairs, wheelchair
Dressing - upper trunk and arms, lower trunk and legs, feet
Personal hygiene - face, hair and arms, trunk and perineum, lower extremities
Bowel and bladder - bowel program, bladder program and catheter care
Feeding

Scoring

Scoring is based on a 3-point ordinal scale:
      D - completely dependent in task
      A or S - requires assistance or supervision
      I - totally independent
Performance on each task is rated and the task ratings in each category are added. A category score is obtained as follows:
      4 - All rated I
      3 - 1 or 2 A/S, all others the client was I
      2 - All other possibilities not covered in 4,3,1,0
      1 - 1 or 2 A/S or 1/I, the rest are D
      0 - All D
Category scores are summed to obtain a total score.

RELIABILITY

Internal consistency

Not reported.

Test-retest Reliability

Not reported.

Interrater Reliability

Forty-three raters scored a series of evaluations. Correlations for the total scores were moderate (0.67-0.74) with the locomotor category rating lower (0.42-0.46).[1]

Six physical therapy students rated videos of evaluations of 6 clients. ICC's were moderate (0.67-0.74).[2]

VALIDITY

Content (domain or face)

Not reported.

Construct

Not reported.

Concurrent

One hundred and forty-eight stroke clients were tested on the Kenny and the Barthel. Correlations were moderate (Kappa .42; r = .73). The Kenny rates more clients as independent compared to the Barthel.

Responsiveness

One study found the Barthel more sensitive to change over time than the Kenny. Another study found the Kenny more sensitive to change than the Barthel and the Katz. No statistical analyses were reported.[3]

IMPORTANT REFERENCES ARE FOUND ON PAGE 186.

A.13. Klein-Bell Activities of Daily Living Scale

DESCRIPTION

The Klein-Bell ADL scale was designed for clinical use, both for planning and evaluating treatment, and for research.[1]

Population	Time to Complete	Cost	Training
Adult clients with any disability.	A maximum of 10 minutes is allowed for each item.	Not indicated.	None required.

INSTRUCTIONS

The items are provided in a list, with little explanation of the administration procedures.

SCALING

Format

Task performance.

Subscales

170 behavioral items are divided into 6 subscales:

Dressing	Bathing/hygiene
Mobility	Eating
Elimination	Emergency Communication

Scoring

Each item is scored on a 2-point nominal scale:

Achieved - performed without verbal or physical assistance from another person
Failed - assistance required

Each item receives a 1, 2 or 3 weighting depending on the difficulty of the item, the time required to perform the item and how critical the skill is to one's health.

The points for each item completed independently in each skill area are summed and are then combined to give an overall ADL independence score.

RELIABILITY

Internal consistency

Not reported.

Test-retest Reliability

Not reported.

Interrater Reliability

Six pairs of raters tested 20 clients with physical disability. 92% agreement was observed.

VALIDITY

Content (domain or face)

Not reported.

Construct

Not reported.

Concurrent

The total score on the Klein-Bell ADL scale correlated with the number of hours per week of assistance required for ADL at 5-10 months post-discharge (determined through phone interview)(-0.86).[2]

Predictive

Not reported.

Responsiveness

Not reported.

IMPORTANT REFERENCES ARE FOUND ON PAGE 187.

A.14. Level of Rehabilitation Scale (LORS-II)

DESCRIPTION

The LORS-II was designed to meet the criteria by the Commission on Accreditation of Rehabilitation Facilities (CARF). It is an instrument for gathering and summarizing functional ratings of clients from hospital-based rehabilitation programs. LORS-II is a substantial revision of the LORS-I. The LORS-II can be used in clinical practice and for research purposes.[1-4]

Population	Time to Complete	Cost	Training
All adult clients in rehabilitation programs, (e.g. head injuries, orthopaedic injuries, stroke, spinal cord injuries, amputations, MS).	Not reported.	None for assessment. Computer time may be a factor.	Some training required.

INSTRUCTIONS

Test manual available.[1]

SCALING

Format

Questionnaire: Nurse and/or therapist rates client on what is known about client performance.

Subscales

The LORS-II is divided into 3 subscales:
ADL - dressing, grooming, washing and bathing, toileting, feeding (10 ratings)
Mobility - walk, wheelchair (2 ratings)
Communication - verbal, gestural, written (8 ratings)
The scale is rated by :
 RN and OT - ADL
 RN and PT - mobility
 RN and Speech - communication
The client is only rated on items he/she is receiving therapy for.

Scoring

Each item is rated on a 5-point ordinal scale (0-4) and the scores are then converted to a percentage score from 0 to 100 (100 - independent).
 0 - Cannot/will not perform the activity
 1 - Requires physical assistance
 2 - Standby assistance
 3 - Special equipment or preparation required
 4 - Performs normally

RELIABILITY

Internal consistency
Not reported.

Test-retest Reliability
Not reported.

Interrater Reliability
Not reported.

VALIDITY

Content (domain or face)
Conforms to the 7 out of 9 relevant points listed by the CARF guide to program evaluation for rehabilitation settings in setting up an evaluation system.

Construct
Not reported.

Concurrent
Not reported.

Predictive
Not reported.

Normative data on ADL function are provided for stroke clients 65 and 75 years of age at admission and discharge with 127 stroke clients being evaluated to develop the norms. Norms were constructed using a regression equation to relate mean of nurse and OT admission ratings to the mean of 2 discharge ratings. A table is provided giving the percentage of clients expected to be discharged at or above various ADL levels (Multiple r = 0.73).[3]

Responsiveness
Six thousand, one hundred and ninety-four clients in 22 facilities using LORS American Data System (LADS) were tested. Those with a longer length of stay have a greater gain in scores on the LORS-II. A curvilinear relationship between functional status at admission and functional gain was found for several impairment groups. Older clients made less progress. Those most severely disabled at admission had the least gain.[2-5]

IMPORTANT REFERENCES ARE FOUND ON PAGE 187.

A.15. The PULSES Profile

DESCRIPTION

The PULSES was developed to evaluate the functional independence in ADL of the chronically ill and elderly institutionalized population.[1,2] In addition, it is a method of consolidating fragments of clinical information gathered in a rehabilitation setting by various staff members involved in the client's daily care. The PULSES was designed for clinical practice, to help predict rehabilitation potential, evaluate progress, and assist in program planning.

Population	Time to Complete	Cost	Training
All clients with physically disabling conditions, (e.g. stroke, other neurological disorders, cardiac conditions, burns, lower limb amputations, and the aged infirm).	Not reported.	Minimal.	None required.

INSTRUCTIONS

The items are listed, but little direction for the administration of each item is provided. Each of the scores 1-4 is clearly defined.

SCALING

Format

Task Performance – Interview – Observations.

Subscales

The scale consists of 6 subscales, each tested several aspects of functional ability:
Physical condition (health, illness status)
Upper limb functions (self care - drinking and eating, dressing, donning brace or prosthesis, washing,bathing, perineal care)
Lower limb functions (mobility - transferring, walking, climbing stairs, wheelchair mobility)
Sensory components (sight, communication)
Excretory functions (bladder, bowel)
Support factors (intellectual and emotional adaptability, support from family and financial support)

Scoring

Scoring is based on a 4-point ordinal scale for a maximum score of 24.
1 - independent/intact
4 - fully dependent
Each of the 6 subscores may be presented separately. The subscales are summed to give an overall measure of functional independence.

RELIABILITY

Internal consistency

Not reported.

Test-retest Reliability

The Granger adapted version (1979) was evaluated for test-retest reliability. A high correlation was found (0.87).[3]

Interrater Reliability

The Granger adapted version (1979) was studied for interrater agreement. The correlation for the total score was extremely high (>.95).[3]

VALIDITY

Content (domain or face)

Not reported.

Construct

Not reported.

Concurrent

One hundred clients, aged 16 to 76 years of age were tested on the Granger adapted version of the PULSES and the Barthel. The correlation between the total scores was moderate (-.65), correlations for the individual subscales varied considerably (-.06 to -.79) with the weakest correlations for the physical condition and the support factors subscales.[3]

Predictive

Not reported.

Responsiveness

Three hundred and seven severely disabled adults from 10 rehabilitation centers were tested at home. The PULSES is capable of measuring change from admission to discharge to follow-up at 2 years for different diagnostic groups.

Discharge scores for those returning home were lower (more independent) than those who were living in long-term care institutions, which in turn were lower than those of clients in acute care. The test does not measure as discrete functions as the Barthel (i.e. eating, ambulation).

IMPORTANT REFERENCES ARE FOUND ON PAGE 188.

A.16. Rivermead Motor Assessment (RMA)

DESCRIPTION

The RMA is an evaluation used to measure physical recovery and progress following stroke.[1-5] It has been more recently developed into The Rivermead Mobility Index; a measure of mobility ranging from bedbound to running, including both fundamental mobility (independent of choice, culture or class) and elective mobility (undertaken entirely by positive choice). The RMA is used clinically as a basis for treatment and as a record of progress during rehabilitation.

Population	Time to Complete	Cost	Training
Stroke clients, developed on adults younger than 65 years.	Less than 30 minutes.	Minimal.	None required.

INSTRUCTIONS
A short definition of each item is described.

SCALING

Format

> Task Performance.
> Questionnaire (has been used with gross function scale).

Subscales

> The test consists of 38 items divided into three subtests:
> > Gross function - functional movement (13 items)
> > Leg and trunk function - control of movement (10 items)
> > Arm function - control and functional movement of arm (15 items)

Scoring

> Each item is scored on a 2-point nominal scale
> > 1 - performed item
> > 0 - did not perform item

RELIABILITY

Internal consistency

Not reported.

Test-retest Reliability

Twenty stroke clients (2 to 6 years post-stroke) aged 48 to 82 years were evaluated twice within 3 weeks on the RMA. Kappa results were poor (total: 0.23; individual items: 0.33 - 0.37). A second study evaluated test-retest reliability on 10 stroke clients, resulting in moderate to high correlations (0.66 - 0.93).[1]

Interrater Agreement

Seven raters evaluating stroke clients found no significant differences in resultant scores on the gross motor function, leg and trunk subscales. However, a significant difference between one rater and the remaining six was found on the arm function subscale.[1]

VALIDITY

Content (domain or face)

Not reported.

Construct

Fifty-one stroke clients, aged 17-65 years were evaluated on the RMA. A strong Guttman scale was found for all three subscales (strong coefficient of scalability: 0.79 - 0.96).[1]

Concurrent

The RMA and the Barthel were used to evaluate 53 stroke clients upon admission to a rehabilitation ward, and at one month and one year later. Correlations ranged from moderate to high for the total score (0.63 - 0.85) and were more variable for the individual subscales (0.38 - 0.85).[2]

Predictive

Not reported.

Responsiveness

Not reported.

IMPORTANT REFERENCES ARE FOUND ON PAGE 189.

A.17. Rivermead ADL Assessment

DESCRIPTION

The Rivermead ADL assessment evaluates the recovery of activities of daily living skills for clients following stroke. The Rivermead ADL assessment was designed to be used both clinically and for research purposes.[1,2]

Population	Time to Complete	Cost	Training
The assessment was developed on adult stroke clients. It has also been used with head injured clients.	Not indicated.	Not indicated.	None required.

INSTRUCTIONS

A short description of each item is provided.

SCALING

Format
Task Performance.

Subscales
The assessment consists of 3 subscales:
Self care (16 items)
Household 1 (9 items)
Household 2 (6 items)

Scoring
Scoring is based on a 3-point ordinal scale:
1 - dependent
2 - independent, requires verbal supervision
3 - independent, with/without aid

RELIABILITY

Internal consistency

Not reported.

Test-retest Reliability

Ten stroke clients at least 6 months post-stroke were evaluated twice within 4 weeks. Correlation between the scores was high (0.95).[1]

Interrater Reliability

Evaluations of 15 clients were scored by 3 raters. Kendall coefficients were high (0.84 - 0.89).[1]

VALIDITY

Content (domain or face)

Not reported.

Construct

The items on the Rivermead ADL assessment form a moderately strong Guttman scale (Coefficient of scalibility: 0.68 - 0.92).[1] The assessment was evaluated for an elderly population with resultant coefficients of scalibility ranging from 0.79 - 0.93.[2]

Concurrent

Not reported.

Predictive

Not reported.

Responsiveness

Not reported.

IMPORTANT REFERENCES ARE FOUND ON PAGE 189.

A.18. The Functional Autonomy Measurement System (SMAF)

DESCRIPTION

The SMAF is used to measure the level of independence in individuals with disabilities and handicaps. It was designed as a global evaluative instrument according to the WHO classification of impairment, disability, and handicap.[1,2] The SMAF was designed to help allocate appropriate community services or chronic care beds to the elderly population.

Population	Time to Complete	Cost	Training
The elderly with all ranges of handicap and disability.[3]	Average of 42 minutes.	Scoring sheets must be purchased.	None required.

INSTRUCTIONS

General directions for the administration and scoring of each item is provided.

SCALING

Format

> Task Performance.
> Interview.

Subscales

> The SMAF is composed of 29 items divided into 5 fundamental areas of functional abilities: (These items are closely related to the WHO classification for disabilities):
>> Activities of Daily Living: eating, bathing, dressing, grooming, urinary continence, fecal continence, using the bathroom.
>> Mobility: transfers, walking around, walking outside, putting on prosthesis or orthosis, moving around in a wheelchair, using the stairs.
>> Communications: seeing, hearing, talking.
>> Mental functions: memory, orientation, understanding, judgement, behaviour.
>> Instrumental activities of daily living: cleaning the house, preparing meals, shopping, doing the laundry, using the phone, using public transportation, taking medication, managing the budget.

Scoring

> Each item is scored on a 4-point ordinal scale:
>> 0 - Complete autonomy
>> 1 - Requires surveillance or stimulation
>> 2 - Requires help
>> 3 - Total dependence
>
> Each item on the scale is verified as to whether the respondent's social and material resources compensate for the disability. If so, the handicap is zero; if not, the handicap becomes proportional to the disability. The evaluator also describes the resource as well as its short-term stability.

RELIABILITY

Internal consistency

Not reported.

Test-retest Reliability

A random sample of 146 elderly people using home care services or on the waiting list for chronic care beds were evaluated twice within 24 hours by two different evaluators using the SMAF. Evaluators included community and institutional nurses and social workers. Agreement ranged from 68% to 78% and the weighted Kappa was moderate (0.53 to 0.76).[4]

Interrater Reliability

Not reported.

VALIDITY

Content (domain or face)

The SMAF attempted to synthesize items from several scales: Katz ADL, Psychiatric Behavioral Scales, Lawton's Instrumental Activities of Daily Living.

Construct

Not reported.

Concurrent

The information obtained on the SMAF was compared to a validated measure of nursing care time. Nine items were eliminated for this study since the nursing care measure could only be used with chronic care clients. Ninety-nine clients, representing the total range of the disability scale, were evaluated. Correlations between the two scales ranged from poor to good (0.58 - 0.89; ADL 0.89, Mobility 0.83, Communication 0.58, Mental functions 0.63).[4]

Predictive

Not reported.

Responsiveness

The SMAF was shown to distinguish the functional abilities of residents of old age homes, nursing homes and long-term care institutions. Residents of the old age homes had lower (more autonomous) scores than those in nursing homes, and lower than those in the long-term care institutions.[5]

IMPORTANT REFERENCES ARE FOUND ON PAGE 189.

A.19.   Patient Evaluation Conference System (PECS)

DESCRIPTION

The PECS tracks small changes in functional performance throughout a dynamic rehabilitation program. It measures a broad spectrum of areas and is interdisciplinary in approach.[1-3] The form documents functional status, as well as evaluating progress toward goals for rehabilitation. The scale is simple to administer, score and interpret. Each of the scales are uniform in interpretation. The evaluation is also adaptable to computer. The PECS is used both clinically to set client goals and measure progress, and for research purposes.

Population	Time to Complete	Cost	Training
All rehabilitation diagnostic groups.	Not reported.	None.	None required.

INSTRUCTIONS

Specific instructions for each of the items are not provided.

SCALING

Format

Observation - Questionnaire.

Subscales

The evaluations system includes a total of 79 items, divided into the following subscales:

Rehabilitation Medicine	Assistive Devices
Rehabilitation Nursing	Psychological
Physical Mobility (7 items)	Social
Activities of Daily Living (6 items)	Vocational-Educational
Communication	Recreation
Medications	Pain
Nutrition	Pulmonary Rehabilitation

Scoring

Each section is scored by the staff member who has primary responsibility for that aspect of care. The sections are then collated onto a master form summarizing the rehabilitation caseload. Each item is scored on an 8-point ordinal scale:

0 - not measured or unable to measure
1 - most dependent
4 - dependent with minor assistance
5 - independent with self-help aids
7 - independent

The clients' current status is marked with an X, and the goal for each item is marked with an O. The form is designed so that each item is examined separately for evidence of rehabilitation progress or goal attainment.

RELIABILITY

Internal consistency

Not reported.

Test-retest Reliability

Not reported.

Interrater Reliability

One hundred and twenty-five clients were evaluated. Correlations between raters were moderate (0.68 - 0.80).[3]

VALIDITY

Content (domain or face)

Confirmed by discussion at client conferences.

Construct and Concurrent

Not reported.

Predictive

Thirty-two traumatic brain injury clients, aged 16-55 were tested a median of 5.3 weeks from injury. The Adaptive Physical Functioning (APF) was performed at discharge. The PECS was poorly predictive of motor loss ($r = 0.61$) and joint limitations ($r = 0.50$). When 204 clients were tested upon admission and at discharge from a rehabilitation center, the initial score was predictive of the final score 53-67% of the time, and was within 1 score 80 - 83% of the time.[4]

Brief Symptom Inventory (BSI) - Level of distress and PECS. N = 40, 22 responders >16 year brain injury 1-11 years after.[5]

$r = -.465$ p $>.083$

Significant:	- self care	Non - Significant:	- recreation
	- mobility		- education
	- living arrangements		- employment
	- communication		

Responsiveness

Not reported.

IMPORTANT REFERENCES ARE FOUND ON PAGE 190.

A.20.   The Canadian Neurological Scale (CNS)

DESCRIPTION

To evaluate and monitor neurological status in conscious and aphasic clients. It is a standardized method of assessing central nervous system dysfunction in clients who are alert or drowsy following a stroke and to detect clinically noteworthy differences in neurological status in the acute stages of stroke. It is a quick and simple method and may be used and interpreted by a variety of professional observers. The Canadian Neurological Scale was designed for clinical use.

Population	Time to Complete	Cost	Training
Acute phase of stroke, all ages.	Less than 5 minutes.	A few simple objects are required.	Designed to be administered by neurologists and physical therapists.

INSTRUCTIONS

Detailed instructions for the administration and the scoring of each item are provided.[1,2]

SCALING

Format

Task performance.

Subscales

I.   Mentation - (maximum 7 points): Level of consciousness, orientation, speech.

II.A1. Motor Function - Weakness, (maximum 11.5 points): (For those with no comprehension defect): Face. Arm: proximal, arm: distal. Leg: proximal, leg: distal.

II.A2. Motor Response - (maximum 3.5 points): (For those with comprehension defect): Face, arms, legs.

Scoring

The items are scored on a variable ordinal scale. Each level of each item is weighted according to the relative importance of the particular neurological deficit, under examination. Weights vary from 0 through 3 by 0.5.

RELIABILITY

Internal consistency

Two studies[1,2] were performed evaluating the scale's internal consistency. When 129 assessments of 34 stroke clients aged 20-87 years were observed by 3 to 4 evaluators (nurse and neurologist), Cronbach's alpha indicated a high level of reliability (.9-1.0). One hundred and fifty-five clients were also tested with a slightly lower resultant reliability (0.79).

Test-retest Reliability

Not reported.

Interrater Reliability

Thirty-four stroke clients aged 20-87 years were tested by 3 or 4 observers using the Canadian Neurological Scale. Kappa ranged from moderate to high (.54-1.00). A second study evaluated 144 clients twice, with an average of 1.63 hours separating the evaluations. Kappa ranged from poor to high (0.54-0.84) for the individual items, and the correlation for the total score was high (0.92).[1]

VALIDITY

Content (domain or face)

The CNS was validated by a panel of experts who agreed on the items to be included and their respective weights.[2]

Construct

Not reported.

Concurrent

One hundred and fifty-five clients were tested an average interval between the initial CNS evaluation and the neurologic examination of 3.7 hours. Correlations between the tests were moderate (.57-.78).[1]

Predictive

The outcomes of 157 stroke clients were examined according to their results in the Canadian Neurological Scale.[1]
    1. Death at 6 months: CNS 11:2.1%, CNS < 9:13.2%
    2. Vascular event within 6 months: CNS 11:2.1%, CNS <9:20.6%
    3. Independent in ADL at 5 months.
High initial CNS scores related to favourable outcomes.

Responsiveness

The scores on the CNS and the Glasgow Coma Scale (GCS) were compared to results of the initial standard neurological examination (SNE). Correlations between the CNS and the SNE were moderate (0.77) but unacceptable between the GCS and SNE (0.56) for 79 neurological ICU clients.

IMPORTANT REFERENCES ARE FOUND ON PAGE 191.

A.21. Clinical Outcome Variable Scale (COVS)

DESCRIPTION

The Clinical Outcome Variable Scale (COVS) is a modification of the physical mobility items from the PECS with the addition of four items from the CPA Health Status Rating Scale[1] and additional items developed to meet the needs of adult rehabilitation clients receiving physiotherapy.

Population	Time to Complete	Cost	Training
Rehabilitation clients receiving physiotherapy.	None indicated.	None indicated.	None indicated.

INSTRUCTIONS

Specific guidelines are available from Louise Seaby, The Rehabilitation Centre, 505 Smyth, Ottawa, ON, K1H 8M2.

SCALING

Format

Task performance.

Subscales

The 11 item mobility subscale includes: rolling (2), lying to sitting balance, transfers (2), ambulation (4), and wheelchair mobility. There are 2 items for arm function.

Scoring

A 7-point ordinal scale is used
   1 - dependent
   2 - assistance
   4 - supervision
   7 - normal

RELIABILITY

Intrarater Reliability

Exact agreement was high (85 to 96%), weighted kappa 0.79 - 0.98. Spearman correlation 0.79 - 0.99. Confidence interval 0.76 - 0.83 to 0.92 - 0.99. The modified version of the physical mobility scale was used for the evaluation of interrater reliability. Twenty-eight physical therapists evaluated a total of 100 clients (20 clients in each of 5 units spinal cord, amputee, stroke, neurolocomotor, outpatient). The interval between the two testing times was 24-48 hours.

Internal consistency

The modified version of the physical mobility scale was used in the item analysis. Cronbach's alpha was used for the combination of 12 items. The item to total correlations ranged from 0.65 - 0.85 with two arm function items having values of 0.30 and 0.34.[2]

Interrater Agreement

After removal of one item that demonstrated poor internal consistency an ICC of 0.97 was found. Confidence Interval = 0.63 - 0.69 to 0.94 - 0.99

VALIDITY

Content (domain or face)

Based on items from other measures with good content validity and additional items developed by health care providers in rehabilitation setting.

Concurrent

Is reported as high in relation to mobility items in the Health Status Rating Form and the Kenny Self-Care Evaluation.[2]

Predictive

Not reported.

Responsiveness

Not reported.

IMPORTANT REFERENCES ARE FOUND ON PAGE 191.

B.1.   Visual Analogue Scale (VAS)

DESCRIPTION

Gradually adopted as a means of quantifying the subjective measure of pain, it is most commonly used as a treatment outcome measure, both clinically and in research. The VAS measures the intensity or magnitude of pain along a continuous scale. It consists of a straight line, usually 100 mm in length. The ends are defined in terms of the extreme limits of the pain experience, no pain and the worst pain ever experienced. The orientation of this line can be either vertical or horizontal. There are 2 types of VAS, absolute and comparative. The absolute measures the severity of the pain at a particular point in time, while the comparative gives a measure of pain relief over time. It is a continuous scale meant to measure the magnitude or intensity of pain or pain relief. Other uses, such as measuring degree of disability, have been studied but were not considered here.

Population	Time to Complete	Cost	Training
Back pain, cancer, rheumatoid arthritic and chronic pain populations.	Explanation and administration of task < 5 min. scoring < 1 min.	Photocopy costs.	None required.

INSTRUCTIONS

The instructions are outlined in the literature and are quite straight forward. It is important that these instructions be clearly communicated to the individual. It is recommended that its use be carefully considered for the elderly population, whose abstracting ability may be impaired. The reliability and validity have been noted to drop considerably in individuals with perceptual problems or impaired motor co-ordination.

SCALING

Format

Self-report.

Subscales

None.

Scoring

The number of millimetres from the no pain line is measured. Precautions should be taken to prevent distortion of the 100 mm line during repeated photocopying, as this may affect the results.

RELIABILITY

Internal consistency

Not reported.

Test-retest Reliability

In a study looking at the reproducibility of the VAS, it was found that reproducibility varies along the length of the line. The lowest reproducibility occurs plus or minus 20mm from the mid-point of the line according to Dixon.[1] That study used a low number of subjects (n=8) and therefore these results should not be considered definitive. Reproducibility has also been reported with an r = 0.99 at the p < 0.05 level.[2]

Intrarater Reliability

Not applicable for self-report scales.

Interrater Reliability

Not applicable for self-report scales.

VALIDITY

Content (domain or face)

The VAS directly measures the intensity of pain and therefore has high content validity.

Construct

Construct validity cannot be assured as there is no clear operational definition of pain. It would be difficult to determine if the intended construct is being measured or if some other construct, i.e. anxiety is being factored in. The VAS assumes that pain is a linear entity. Due to the linear nature and the fixed length of the line, floor and ceiling effects are problematic.

Concurrent

The VAS and the Numeric Pain Rating Scale have a correlation ranging from r = 0.77 to 0.91.[3] The correlation between the VAS and the finger dynamometer was r = 0.87 (p = 0.001).[4] The finger dynamometer is a device that registers the amount of force exerted that the individual believes is comparable to the pain intensity. Between the VAS and a verbal description scale of pain, a correlation of r = 0.81 to 0.87 (p = 0.01-0.001) was found.[4]

Predictive

Not reported

Responsiveness

In developing the VAS it was found that individuals are able to detect 21 levels of just noticeable differences (JND) between the initial detection of pain and intolerable pain.[5] It is felt that these 21 levels are detectable using the VAS. It is felt by some that the VAS is less sensitive to change in acute than in chronic pain.[6,7]

IMPORTANT REFERENCES ARE FOUND ON PAGE 191.

B.2.   Numeric Pain Rating Scale (NPRS)

DESCRIPTION

The NPRS (developer unknown) is a numeric scale to measure the magnitude or intensity of pain. The individual is asked to select a number to represent the intensity of the pain at the moment. The scale is 0-10, with 0 being no pain and 10 being the worst pain imaginable. It can be administered either verbally or in written form.

The NPRS was developed as a means of quantifying the subjective measure of pain. It is commonly used as a treatment outcome measure, both clinically and in research.[1,2]

Population	Time to Complete	Cost	Training
Individuals with low back pain as well as rheumatoid arthritis and cancer.[3]	Explanation and administration: 5 min.	No cost.	None required.

INSTRUCTIONS

The instructions are very straight forward. It is important that these instructions be communicated clearly to the individual.

SCALING

Format
   Self-report.

Subscales
   None.

Scoring
   The examiner documents the value reported by the individual.

RELIABILITY

Internal consistency
Not reported.

Test-retest Reliability
Not reported.

Interrater Reliability
N/A.

VALIDITY

Content (domain or face)
The NPRS directly measures the intensity of pain and therefore has high content validity.

Construct
Construct validity cannot be assured as there is no clear operational definition of pain and even with a clear definition, it would be difficult to determine if the intended construct is being measured or if some other construct, i.e. anxiety, is included.[4]

Concurrent
The NPRS and the VAS were found to have a correlation of $r = 0.80$ ($p < 0.01$). The NPRS and the finger dynamometer showed a correlation of 0.47 to 0.68 ($p < 0.01$). The finger dynamometer is a device that registers the amount of force exerted by the individual's finger comparable to the individual's pain intensity.

Predictive
Not reported.

Responsiveness
Not reported.

IMPORTANT REFERENCES ARE FOUND ON PAGE 192.

B.3.   Pain Drawing

DESCRIPTION

Developed by Ransford, Cairns, and Mooney[1] with scoring modified slightly by Schwartz and DeGood[2] and further by Margolis, Tait, and Krause,[3] the pain drawing is a screening test to determine whether or not further psychological evaluation is required. The pain drawing can be successfully used for improving communication between clients and clinicians and summarizes the subjective information concerning pain location. It is also used as a component of a diagnostic battery to aid in establishing individual treatment programs and later used to assess treatment outcome. It also has its place in research as an outcome measure for evaluating the effectiveness of treatment programs. The pain drawing assesses the location of the pain and the presence or absence of non-anatomical pain representation. The pain drawing consists of two body outlines, front and back. The non-anatomical pain representation is seen as psychological involvement in the pain pattern.

Population	Time to Complete	Cost	Training
Acute and chronic low back pain.	Including time to give the instructions <5 min. Scoring: up to 5 min.	Photocopy costs.	None required.

INSTRUCTIONS

The individual is asked to draw on the body outlines, areas of pain, numbness and pins and needles. The scoring instructions are found in the literature (see References).

SCALING

Format

Self-report.

Scoring

The original scoring system used a penalty point system.[1] Penalty points were assigned to each drawing based an various characteristics of the drawing. This scoring system was modified to a 5-point Likert scale by rating the drawing on a scale of 1-5 for appropriateness, 1 being completely appropriate and 5 being completely inappropriate. The scoring was later modified by scoring the presence or absence of pain in each of 45 body areas.[2,3]

RELIABILITY

Internal consistency

Because of the large area of the body unaffected by pain, the average percentage of agreement across areas of pain was also calculated. The agreement found was 76.3%.[4]

Test-retest Reliability

Using the surface area method of scoring, a Pearson product-moment correlation coefficient of r = 0.85 at the p < 0.001 level was found by Margolis et al.[4]

Interrater Reliability

Using the penalty point system, correlation coefficients of r = 0.94-0.97 were found. One study[2] found exact agreement between raters in 90% (18/20) of cases.

VALIDITY

Content (domain or face)

The extent to which the pain drawing can isolate pain due to pathologic sources and pain due to psychological involvement is disputed. Many authors feel that the pain drawing is a good indicator of psychologic involvement while others do not. Regardless of the source of pain, the pain drawing is able to identify the location of the pain.

Construct

Its use as a screening test is based on the construct that psychological involvement in pain patterns can be identified by the pain drawing.

Concurrent

Concurrent validity was explored by comparing the pain drawing to the Minnesota Multiphasic Personality Inventory (MMPI), specifically the hysteria (Hy) and hypochondriasis (Hs) scales. It was found that the pain drawings correlated well with the MMPI[5]. Overall association of pain drawing and the MMPI was found to be 89%.[1]

Predictive

When determining the strength of the pain drawing as a predictor of psychological involvement, a value of r = 0.48 (p <0.001) was found.[6] As mentioned earlier, its predictive strength is poor as the sensitivity (number of true positives identified expressed as a percent of the total positives) has been noted to be as low as 42%.[7] Its predictive value for determining psychological involvement is at best questionable with ranges in accuracy of prediction (sensitivity) found between 42% and 93%.[8]

Responsiveness

Not reported.

IMPORTANT REFERENCES ARE FOUND ON PAGE 192.

B.4.   Sickness Impact Profile (SIP)

DESCRIPTION

The SIP was developed as a measure of perceived health status and as an outcome measure of health care across types and severity of illness and across demographic and cultural subgroups by Bergner and Bobbitt;[1-3] Deyo (modified version);[4-7] and Roland and Morris (modified version) (see Disability Questionnaire). It consists of 136 items that fall into 12 categories and 2 dimensions, the physical and the psychosocial. Each item describes a specific dysfunctional behaviour. Deyo[5] modified the measure for use with the LBP population by deleting the categories of eating and communication. In the modified version for low back pain the following categories, are measured: ambulation, mobility, body care and movement, social interaction, alertness, emotional behaviour, sleep and rest, work, home management and recreation and pastime activities. It has been translated into Spanish and the translated version tested for its reliability and validity.[6] The SIP was designed as an outcome measure to be used both clinically and in research, and the attributes examined are extensive.

Population	Time to Complete	Cost	Training
Low back pain.	20-30 minutes for questionnaire. Scoring: 5-10 min with calculator.	Instrument instruction manual less than $10. Other costs: photocopying.	None required.

INSTRUCTIONS

An interviewers' manual and the instrument itself may be obtained from M. Bergner or B Gilson, Dept. of Health Services, School of Public Health and Community Medicine SC-37 University of Washington Seattle, Washington 98195. Respondents are asked to check the items which apply to them on that particular day and are related to their LBP.

SCALING

Format

May be done with either the self-reporting or interviewer format. An adequate level of literacy is required for the self-reporting format.

Subscales

Physical and psychosocial.

Scoring

Items checked are counted and the weighted total of each category is calculated. This sum is divided by the maximum possible score of the SIP and multiplied by 100 to give a total SIP score. Physical and psychosocial dimensions are calculated from the appropriate categories.

RELIABILITY

Internal consistency

Internal consistency was demonstrated between the 2 dimensions, physical and psychosocial (r = 0.85-0.88).[4] Between the individual categories, internal consistency ranged from r = 0.62-0.97 at the p <0.01 level.[1,7]

Test-retest Reliability

A number of authors examined test-retest reliability. The values found for the reliability of the total scores were r = 0.73-0.92.[3,4,6,8] When examining the reliability of the actual items scored, the values were slightly lower, r = 0.45-0.89.[3,8]

Interrater Reliability

Interrater reliability was reported as high.[2] Overall scores did not appear to be affected by different interviewers.[9]

VALIDITY

Content (domain or face)

Content validity is high. The modification made by Deyo helps to improve content validity for people with low back pain, by eliminating the categories of eating and communication.

Construct

Demonstration of the relationship between sickness impacts and behavioral dysfunction.[9] The SIP and self-perceived dysfunction scales had an r = 0.69 value. The SIP and the self-perceived sickness scales had an r = 0.54-0.63 and the SIP and the clinician-perceived dysfunction scales had an r = 0.40-0.52.[1-3] The SIP scores were found to have a positive correlation with "down time" and a negative correlation to "up time".[9] Deyo[5,7] compared the SIP scores to physical observations. The Spearman Correlations results are summarized below:

	SIP[7]	SIP[5]
# of prior episodes	0.28	0.22
spinal flexion	0.48	0.30
straight leg raising	-0.29	-0.18
nerve root irritation	0.29	—
self-rated pain	0.31	0.38

Concurrent

In the comparison of the SIP and the National Health Interview Survey, a correlation of r = 0.55-0.61 was found between the SIP and the Daily Living Index, a correlation of r = 0.46 was found.[3] There was a positive correlation with the psychosocial impairment on the MMPI, reflecting emotional distress.[9]

Predictive: Not reported.

Responsiveness

Deyo[6] reports that the SIP is sensitive to change in the low back pain population as it shows improvement as expected. By using a treatment and control group, Follick et al.[9] showed that the SIP was able to detect a clinically significant change (p <0.01). A percent score change of 27% was found with paired t-tests, significant at the 0.001 level.

IMPORTANT REFERENCES ARE FOUND ON PAGE 193.

B.5.   Disability Questionnaire (DQ)

DESCRIPTION

The Disability Questionnaire is a modification by Roland and Morris[1,2] of the Sickness Impact Profile (SIP). It consists of 24 items. Each item describes a specific dysfunctional behaviour. The items were taken from the SIP with the addition of the phrase, "because of my back". The following attributes are considered: level of activity, body movement, ambulation, activities of daily living, eating and sleeping. It does not measure psychosocial function.[3,4] The DQ was developed as an outcome measure for use both clinically and in research.

Population	Time to Complete	Cost	Training
Back pain population.	Less than 5 minutes are required to complete the questionnaire. Scoring should take less than 2 minutes.	Photocopy costs.	None required.

INSTRUCTIONS

Items are checked if they apply to the respondent on that particular day and are related to the back.

SCALING

Format
May be done with either the interviewer or self-administered format.

Subscales
None.

Scoring
Scoring involves the summing of the positive responses. The scores may range from 0 to 24.

RELIABILITY

Internal consistency

Item agreement percent coefficient was found to be 0.83.[1]

Test-retest Reliability

When examining the total score, a test-retest reliability correlation coefficient was found to be r = 0.91.[1]

Interrater Reliability

Not reported.

VALIDITY

Content (domain or face)

Content validity is less strong than the SIP as the psychosocial domain is excluded from the DQ.

Construct

The DQ shows good agreement with a 6-point pain rating scale.[1] It correlates strongly with the physical dimension of the SIP and has a substantially weaker correlation with the psychosocial dimension as expected.[4]

Concurrent

The DQ correlates well with the SIP (r = 0.85, p <0.001).[4]

Predictive

A high DQ score has been shown to be related to poor outcome (p <0.05), as measured with a global rating scale by health care professionals.[1]

Responsiveness

The DQ was found to be at least as responsive as the full SIP.[3] The DQ change score had a significant association with clinically rated change on a 3-point scale, r = 0.16 at p = 0.05 level.[4] While low, this association is comparable to the correlation between the SIP and the same 3-point scale. It was found to be more sensitive to change than a 6-point pain scale.[1] This may be due to the fact it measures more aspects of disability than simply pain.

IMPORTANT REFERENCES ARE FOUND ON PAGE 194.

B.6.   Oswestry Low Back Pain Disability Questionnaire

DESCRIPTION

Developed by Fairbanks, Davies, Couper, O'Brien, Jones and Hunt at the Orthopaedic Hospital, Oswestry, Shropshire, England, this Questionnaire was meant to quantify the degree of functional impairment of individuals with low back pain. The Oswestry covers 10 different areas of activities of daily living. These include pain, personal care, lifting, walking, sitting, standing, sleeping, sex life, social life and travelling. Each section has 6 statements about the particular activity. Each of the 6 statements represents a different level of severity of disability. The Oswestry has been used for screening, treatment planning, and evaluation of treatment. It is used as an outcome measure in research evaluating the effectiveness of treatment programs. It has been used to examine the relationship between subjective reports of disability and various objective physical findings.

Population	Time to Complete	Cost	Training
Low back pain.	About 3.5-5 min to complete and 2-3 min to score.	Photocopy costs.	No special training required .

INSTRUCTIONS

The instructions are very straightforward and are presented in the article by Fairbanks et al.[1] It is to be presented on pink paper as it has been shown that the pink colour makes the questionnaire more accepting to clients than white.[1]

SCALING

Format
Self-administered questionnaire.

Subscales
None.

Scoring
Each section is scored on a 0-5 scale, 5 representing the greatest disability. The scores of each section are added together for a total score of 50. This number is multiplied by two to get a percent score. This value represents the percentage disability.

RELIABILITY

Internal consistency

Good internal consistency was shown in 22 clients with chronic low back pain. The mean scores of the individual sections correlated with those of the pain section.

Test-retest Reliability

Excellent test-retest reliability was shown with 22 clients with chronic low back pain. A correlation coefficient of $r = 0.99$ was found ($p < 0.001$).[1]

Interrater Reliability

None reported.

VALIDITY

Content (domain or face)

The content validity is fair-poor. The questionnaire is intended to assess disability yet it addresses disability based primarily on pain.

Construct

The questionnaire was developed to measure the level of disability. Fairbanks et al.[1] defined disability as "the limitation of a client's performance compared with that of a fit person". The construct validity is fair as the questionnaire addresses the specific issues that may affect an individual with low back pain but fails to allow for alternate causes of the disability other than pain.

Concurrent

An attempt was made to investigate the concurrent validity of the questionnaire with 25 clients who were suffering from their first attack of low back pain. It was felt that in this group of individuals there was a strong likelihood of spontaneous recovery. The questionnaire was administered at weekly intervals. The gradual improvement that was seen through evaluation of a health care professional, was reflected in the significant change of the Oswestry score over the 3 weeks ($p < 0.005$).[1]

Predictive

Not reported.

Responsiveness

In the study described above,[1] there were significantly different scores ($p < 0.005$), after 3 weeks had elapsed.

IMPORTANT REFERENCES ARE FOUND ON PAGE 194.

B.7. Partial Sit-up/Curl-up as a Test of Abdominal Muscle Strength/Endurance

DESCRIPTION

This protocol based on Faulkner, Sprigings, McQuarrie and Bell[1] is meant to measure the muscular endurance of the abdominal muscles. There are many versions of the partial sit-up/curl-up. Traditionally the one-minute sit-up was used. Essentially this involved counting how many sit-ups an individual could perform in one minute. Quinney felt that this was not an appropriate test for either abdominal muscle strength or endurance.[2] A new protocol was developed and is currently used and advocated in the Canadian Standardized Test of Fitness (CSTF). It is used as part of a battery of tests to assess physical capacity. It is a clinical outcome measure.

Population	Time to Complete	Cost	Training
Normal individuals and back injured population.	10 minutes.	A tape measure, stop watch and metronome.	None required.

INSTRUCTIONS
The individual is asked to do a curl-up by sliding their hand along a tape measure. They must maintain a cadence of 25 curl-ups/minute. The amount of time the individual can maintain the cadence or the number of curl-ups is recorded.

SCALING
Format Task performance. **Subscales** None. **Scoring** Scoring can either be done by recording the number of curl-ups performed, up to maximum of 75 or by recording the amount of time the individual can maintain the cadence, up to a maximum of 3 minutes.

RELIABILITY

Internal consistency

N/A.

Test-retest Reliability

Not reported.

Interrater Reliability

Not reported.

VALIDITY

Content (domain or face)

Content validity for the partial sit-up or curl-up is higher that the full sit-up. The full sit-up involves the hip flexors to a great extent, thus confounding the test.[3] This protocol shows clear floor and ceiling effects.[1]

Construct

EMG studies have confirmed that it is the rectus abdominis and external oblique muscles that are working during a curl-up.[3,4]

Concurrent

Discriminant

Differences have been shown between age groups and between genders within age groups.[1]

Predictive

The partial curl-up is used by the CSTF as part of a battery of tests to assess physical capacity but individually the test has not been shown to have predictive properties.

Responsiveness

Not reported.

IMPORTANT REFERENCES ARE FOUND ON PAGE 194.

B.8. Sorensen Test for Endurance of the Back Musculature

DESCRIPTION

The test developed by Biering-Sorensen measures the muscular endurance of the back extensors. It involves measuring how many seconds the individual can keep the unsupported back horizontal. The Sorensen test is used as a predictor of the occurrence of low back pain. It is also used as an outcome measure, both clinically and in research.

Population	Time to Complete	Cost	Training
Normal population and back injured individuals.	Less than 5 minutes.	Stopwatch and 3 straps.	No special training is required.

INSTRUCTIONS

The individual is prone on a plinth with the trunk hanging over the edge. The legs are firmly strapped to the plinth. The individual is asked to maintain the trunk in a horizontal position for as long a period as possible.

SCALING

Format

Task performance.

Subscales

None.

Scoring

The time that the individual can maintain the position is recorded in seconds.

RELIABILITY

Internal consistency

N/A.

Test-retest Reliability

Scores between tests varied from 7% to 10%.[1,2]

Interrater Reliability

Not reported.

VALIDITY

Content (domain or face)

Content validity may be compromised by the limitations of comfort and motivation.

Construct

During testing, surface electrodes were used to monitor the use of the appropriate musculature.[2]

Concurrent

Not reported.

Predictive

Not reported.

Responsiveness

Not reported.

IMPORTANT REFERENCES ARE FOUND ON PAGE 195.

B.9. Pressure Biofeedback (PBF) for Measuring Muscular Endurance of the Transverse Abdominal and Abdominal Oblique Musculature

DESCRIPTION

The pressure biofeedback device of Richardson and Jull[1-4] is a simple pressure transducer consisting of a tri-sectional bag made of non-elastic material and a pressure gauge. The bag is placed in the small of the back. Movement or change in position causes volume changes in the bag that registers on the dial. The PBF unit is used to detect activation of the transverse and oblique abdominal musculature and can be used to determine endurance of these muscles. It has uses as an outcome measure both clinically and in research. It is also useful as a treatment tool.

Population	Time to Complete	Cost	Training
Normal population and individuals with back pain.	5-10 min for client instruction, learning, rest, and performance.	Approximately $170.	None required.

INSTRUCTIONS

The PBF unit is placed in the small of the back, with the individual in crook lying. The individual is asked to press the small of their back down into the bag until the pressure dial reads an increase in pressure of 10-15 mmHg.

SCALING

Format

Task performance.

Subscales

None.

Scoring

A yes/no scale can be used to determine if the correct muscle recruitment was obtained or a single measure of the amount of time a contraction can be maintained.

RELIABILITY

Internal consistency

Not reported.

Test-retest Reliability

Not reported.

Interrater Reliability

Not reported.

VALIDITY

Content (domain or face)

The transverse abdominal and abdominal oblique musculature have a primary stabilizing function in the lumbar spine.[1] This supports the rationale for measuring muscular endurance of these muscles for lumbar stability.

Construct

Correlation between EMG readings of oblique musculature and the readings of the PBF unit were found to have a range of $r = 0.80\text{-}0.91$.[2]

Concurrent

Not reported.

Predictive

Not reported.

Responsiveness

Not reported.

IMPORTANT REFERENCES ARE FOUND ON PAGE 195.

B.10. Modified Schober Method of Measuring Spinal Mobility

DESCRIPTION

The modified Schober method as modified by Moll and Wright[1,2] and further by Williams, Binkley, Bloch et al.[3] was developed as a diagnostic tool for ankylosing spondylitis.[4] It is used as an outcome measure both clinically and in research. It is a skin distraction/attraction method of measuring lumbar forward flexion, backward extension and lateral flexion. It uses a flexible tape measure and the results are recorded in centimetres. The modified Schober is measuring flexion and extension of the spine, independent of hip movement. It is acknowledged that it is susceptible to error due to skin movement occurring in the absence of spinal movement.

Population	Time to Complete	Cost	Training
Clients with low back pain, ankylosing spondylitis and other forms of arthritis.	Less than 2 minutes.	$5 (tape measure).	Knowledge of the anatomical landmarks.

INSTRUCTIONS

The mid-point between both P.S.I.S. is marked. Another mark is made 10 cm cranially to this, and another mark is made 5 cm caudally to the original mark. The distance between the cranial and caudal marks is measured in the fully flexed and extended positions. A further modification was developed by Williams et al.[3] and is well explained in their article.

SCALING

Format

Task performance.

Subscales

N/A.

Scoring

The distance between anatomical landmarks in the flexed or extended position is subtracted from the original 15 cm.

RELIABILITY

Internal consistency: N/A.

Test-retest Reliability

In 10 subjects with no back pain gave a coefficient of variation (CV) of flexion 0.9% and extension 2.8%.[5] Portek[6] reported forward flexion gave a CV of 8.5% in individuals with no history of LBP. Reynolds[7] showed poor intra-rater reliability (CV of 11.65% in flexion, 21.57% in extension) in a mixed population of individuals with arthritis and others with no LBP. Beattie[8] reported an intraclass correlation (ICC) for extension of 0.93 in 100 individuals with LBP and an ICC of 0.90 for a group with no LBP. Using their re-modified technique in individuals with LBP Williams et al[3] found correlations of r = 0.83-0.89 for flexion and for extension, r = 0.69-0.91.

Interrater Reliability

Interrater agreement was poor in a group with no LBP (p <0.01).[6] In 11 individuals with no LBP, interrater reliability was shown to have an ICC of 0.94.[7] Pile,[9] measuring interrater reliability in individuals with ankylosing spondylitis, by calculating the coefficient of reliability, found it was 0.78 (p=0.007). Miller[10] found a correlation of r = 0.71 in individuals with no LBP. Reynolds[7] showed a correlation coefficient of r = 0.59 in flexion and r = 0.75 (p <0.05) in extension. Williams[3] found ICC of 0.72 for measuring flexion and, using their re-modified technique, 0.76 for extension.

VALIDITY

Content (domain or face)

The technique renders a linear measurement in cm when traditionally joint movement is angular movement, measured in degrees.

Construct

The test is based on the construct that lumbar motion is the sum of the movements taking place at each of the motion segments. Miller[10] questioned the validity as a variable number of motion segments were covered in the 10 cm mark above the P.S.I.S.

Concurrent

Macrae and Wright[1] investigated concurrent validity by examining the correlation between radiographic measurement of the movement between L1 and the sacrum and the modified Schober technique. A correlation coefficient of r = 0.97 was found, with a standard error of 3.25^0. Portek[6] showed a low correlation, r = 0.43, between biplanar x-rays and the modified Schober.

Discriminant

Beattie[8] showed a different distribution of data between individuals with back pain and those without.

Predictive: Not reported.

Responsiveness

The standard deviation for flexion ranges from 1.29 to 1.51 cm and for extension, 0.76 to 1.09 cm. Therefore changes of less that 1.5 cm are not clinically detectable.

IMPORTANT REFERENCES ARE FOUND ON PAGE 195.

B.11. Leighton Flexometer for Measuring Spinal Mobility

DESCRIPTION

The Leighton flexometer[1] is a device with a gravity dependent needle enclosed in a case and has a strap to attach the device to the body. It measures absolute angular displacement in relation to gravity. The exact joint axis does not have to be identified. The Leighton flexometer can be used for screening, treatment planning, evaluation of treatment and as a research tool. The Leighton flexometer can be used to measure gross lumbar flexion, extension, side flexion and rotation. It has the added versatility of measuring movement of the extremities as well as spinal motion.

Population	Time to Complete	Cost	Training
Normal population and high performance athletes.	2 min.	About $160.	No special training, but brief practice required.

INSTRUCTIONS

The instructions are printed in Leighton's original article[1] as well as some exercise physiology texts. A manual has been referenced in some papers. For flexion and extension, the flexometer is placed in the mid-axillary line. For side flexion and rotation, it is placed on the dorsal aspect of the back, in the mid-line.

SCALING

Format

Task performance.

Subscales

Inherent.

Scoring

The measurement is in degrees. The device has a locking mechanism to allow the tester to lock the pointer at maximum range, thereby allowing the subject to return to the erect position before the value is read from the dial. The dial is marked in 1 degree increments.

RELIABILITY

Internal consistency

N/A.

Test-retest Reliability

Not reported.

Intrarater Reliability

Good intrarater reliability has been found in the normal population and high performance athletes with coefficients with a range of r = 0.83-0.996.

Interrater Reliability

Not reported.

VALIDITY

Content (domain or face)

Content validity is fair. The Leighton flexometer is unable to distinguish hip flexion from lumbar flexion.

Construct

The construct validity is based on measuring angular displacement in degrees. The measurements correspond to the recognized segmental movements of the body. It is measuring the sum of the movements occurring at each of the motion segments.

Concurrent

Not reported for measurement of the back.

Predictive

Not reported.

Responsiveness

Not reported.

IMPORTANT REFERENCES ARE FOUND ON PAGE 1961.

B.12. Inclinometer Method of Measuring Spinal Mobility

DESCRIPTION

The inclinometer developed by Loebl[1] is a gravity dependent device to measure angular displacement. The various protocols in the literature describe the measurement of gross flexion and extension, hip flexion, hip extension, true lumbar flexion and extension and lumbar rotation.[2-7]

Population	Time to Complete	Cost	Training
Low back pain, ankylosing spondylitis and rheumatoid arthritis.	Less than two minutes.	Approximately $160 - inclinometer.	Knowledge of anatomical landmarks, brief practice required.

INSTRUCTIONS

The desired protocol using either 1 or 2 inclinometers can be obtained from the literature.

SCALING

Format

Task performance.

Subscales

Inherent.

Scoring

The values in degrees are read off the dial of the inclinometer. The scale is marked off in increments of one degree. Depending on the value desired, simple mathematical calculation may be required.

RELIABILITY

Internal consistency: N/A

Test-retest Reliability[1-7]

In 9 normal subjects, Loebl[1] reported 4° of variation in repeated measures but it is not clear as to whether or not the testing was blinded. In flexion, CV's have a range of 9.3-33.9% in symptom-free individuals. In extension, the CV=3.6-15.7% and for total sagittal range (TSR) the CV=9.6%. ICC of 0.93 was found for spinal flexion in individuals with LBP. Pearson correlation values for LBP sufferers range was r = 0.13-0.87 for flexion and r = 0.28-0.66 for extension. The double inclinometer method has shown an ICC of 0.86 and correlation coefficients of 0.93-0.95. In another low back pain client population, correlation coefficients of 0.97-0.98 have been reported.

Interrater Reliability

The single inclinometer method in a population with individuals with back pain and those without, rendered ICCs of 0.75-0.76 for flexion and extension. Others reported no statistical significant difference in flexion (t = 1.25), extension (t = 0.72) and TSR (t = 0.42). Others reported correlation coefficients for gross flexion r = 0.94, lumbar flexion r = 0.60-0.84, lumbar extension r = 0.48 and pelvic motion r = 0.86, again in a mixed population. Total combined rotation was found to have an r = 0.75 (p <0.001). Another study found right rotation to have an r = 0.45 and left rotation have an r = 0.89.

VALIDITY

Content (domain or face)

Content validity is good. Both the double and single inclinometer methods are able to distinguish between lumbar and hip motion. This is critical if it is true lumbar movement that is of interest and not the gross amount of flexion achieved.

Construct

The construct validity is based on the construct of measuring angular displacement or amount of spinal curvature of the spine and that spinal movement is the sum of the movement at each motion segment.

Concurrent

Correlation between inclinometer methods and biplanar x-rays show correlation coefficients from 0.42 (in a population of asymptomatic individuals) to 0.76 (in a population with LBP).[8-10] One study showed no statistically significant difference between the double and single inclinometer methods used in a normal population (p <0.01). In a no LBP population, in flexion, the inclinometer and kyphometer had an r = 0.89-0.99, the inclinometer and the flexicurve had an r = 0.94 and the inclinometer and the modified Schober had an r = 0.04. In extension, inclinometer and flexicurve had an r = 0.90 and inclinometer and kyphometer, an r = 0.92.

Predictive: Not reported.

Responsiveness

Not addressed directly. Because SDs for flexion were 8.59-11.56° and for extension, 6.39-10.25°, changes of less than 12° are probably not clinically detectable.

IMPORTANT REFERENCES ARE FOUND ON PAGE 197.

B.13. Lifting Dynamometers

DESCRIPTION

As with the measurement of trunk strength, there are a number of technologies available for measuring lifting capacity. Lifting capacity can be measured isometrically, isokinetically and gravity-inertially. Isometric lifts involve no actual movement: isokinetic lifts have the velocity held constant and the gravity-inertial lifts have the mass held constant.[1] Traditionally, the lifts have been constrained to control as many of the variables as possible. Recently, the Lido Company has produced a Lido Liftask that allows three-dimensional, unconstrained lifting. Testing often involves not only determining a maximum lifting capacity but lifting endurance. The disadvantages of this type of technology is the cost and divergence from the true lifting situations. One advantage is the ability to detect less than maximum effort through looking at the coefficients of variation (CV). Any CV greater than 10% is thought to represent sub-maximal effort.[2,3]

Population	Time to Complete	Cost	Training
Normal population and individuals with back pain.	30-60 minutes.	$50,000-$100,000 including computer and software.	One half day training and 1/2-1 days of practice.

INSTRUCTIONS

Isometric protocols have been developed from the literature while the isokinetic and gravity-inertial protocols have been developed from pilot testing and the real world model. No reliability and validity testing has been published to date.

SCALING

Format

Task performance.

Subscales

Inherent.

Scoring

There are large databases available for the constrained lifting dynamometers. These databases can be compared to the results generated by the computer.

RELIABILITY

Internal consistency

Not reported.

Test-retest Reliability

Not reported.

Interrater Reliability

Not reported.

VALIDITY

Content (domain or face)

The content validity is high in the unconstrained lifting dynamometers as these most effectively simulate real world lifting. The constrained lifting dynamometers have a lower content validity as it is difficult to simulate true to life lifting.

Construct

Not reported.

Concurrent

Not reported.

Predictive

Not reported.

Responsiveness

Not reported.

IMPORTANT REFERENCES ARE FOUND ON PAGE 198.

B.14. Isokinetic Dynamometers

DESCRIPTION

The Cybex Trunk Extension/Flexion and Torso Rotation spinal isokinetic dynamometers are examples of isokinetic devices used to measure spinal muscle strength.[1-3] Other manufacturers have more recently introduced devices with different features. The testing positions are variable as are the types of muscle contractions which can be tested. Therefore, comparisons between studies should be done with caution. A variety of attachments allows use with a number of joints. Trunk rotation is measured with a separate device designed specifically for this task. The isokinetic dynamometers can be used to measure trunk flexion, extension and rotation, both isometrically and isokinetically and can be used to evaluate muscle strength and endurance. The results of testing can be used for treatment planning and as an outcome measure, both clinically and in research.

Population	Time to Complete	Cost	Training
Normal population and individuals with low back pain.	30-60 minutes.	Approximately $18,000 including computer and software.	One half day training and 1-2 days of practice.

INSTRUCTIONS

The manufacturer provides a manual on the use of the Cybex and includes some recommended protocols. The literature also has modified protocols. Testing requires at least 4 maximal flexion/extension performance repetitions at various speeds with rest intervals of 20 sec between repetitions. A 10 min warm-up and practice repetitions precede the testing.

SCALING

Format

Task performance.

Subscales

Inherent.

Scoring

The associated computer provides a printout on the following parameters: peak torque trunk flexion (Nm), peak torque trunk extension (Nm), range at which peak torque is reached (degrees), peak torque as a percent of body weight ratio, peak torque at 30° (Nm), peak torque at 60° (Nm), flexion-extension peak ratio, maximum ROM tested, average ROM, peak total energy acceleration (joules), total energy first 2 and last 2 repetitions (joules), endurance ratio, average power (watts) and work ratio flexion-extension.

RELIABILITY

Internal consistency

N/A

Test-retest Reliability

Pearson correlation coefficients between trials on the same day were r = 0.80-0.99 in flexion and r = 0.88-0.99 in extension. Pearson correlation coefficients between trials on different days were r = 0.76-0.77 in flexion and 0.74-0.96 in extension.

Interrater Reliability

Pearson correlation coefficients are reported r > 0.90.

VALIDITY

Content (domain or face)

Muscle strength measured by the isokinetic dynamometer represents the maximum instantaneous tension in the muscle. In the test described in the literature the torque values recorded include not only the strength of the trunk muscles in the sagittal plane but also the strength of the hip muscles.[2]

Construct

EMG studies have shown that the erector spinae and oblique abdominal musculature are working during trunk rotation.[3]

Concurrent

Trunk rotation and trunk extension strengths correlated moderately well, r = 0.66-0.77. That is to be expected as the same muscles are working in both situations.

Predictive

Not reported.

Responsiveness

Testing showed a substantial increase in strength after a treatment program that was intended to increase strength.

IMPORTANT REFERENCES ARE FOUND ON PAGE 198.

C.1. Heart Rate

DESCRIPTION

One of the vital signs, heart rate is simply a measure of the number of heart beats (cardiac cycles) per minute. It may be measured by an electrocardiogram, an auditory method, a palpation method or by portable heart rate monitors based on the principles of plethysmography.

For the purposes of this report, the focus will be on the palpation technique of heart rate determination. The most common sites for this method are the carotid and radial arteries, palpated with the digits 2 and 3. The number of cycles is usually counted over a 6, 10 or 15 second interval, and multiplied by an appropriate factor to reflect the number of beats per minute.

Population	Time to Complete	Cost	Training
Children and adults; normal or those with suspected or established cardiorespiratory problems.	Less than 1 minute.	Minimal.	None required.

INSTRUCTIONS

There are a multitude of basic text references and guidelines available for the performance of the technique.[1] Ranges of normal resting heart rates vary with position, age and sex and are readily available in any basic text.

SCALING

Format

No active participation is required of the individual being assessed.

Subscales

Inherent.

Scoring

Heart rate is recorded in beats per minute. Values may be used to evaluate response to exercise in accordance with previously reported reference norms (based on the known linearity of the relationship between heart rate and oxygen consumption, VO_2).

RELIABILITY

Internal consistency
Not available.

Interrater Reliability
No data found.

Interrater Reliability
Not reported.

VALIDITY

Content (domain or face)
Inherent.

Construct
The relationship between heart rate and exercise intensity is known and accepted and is classically described in Astrand and Rodahl's text.[2]

The accuracy of post-exercise heart rate as a reflection of exercise intensity has been the subject of much investigation. There is general agreement that if the heart rate is measured within 15 seconds of the conclusion of exercise that it will provide a valid indicator (being less than 4% lower) of intensity during exercise in normal individuals.[3-6]

There is controversy about whether measuring the carotid pulse versus the radial pulse introduces error to the measurement by virtue of the possible stimulation of the carotid sinus reflex.

Concurrent
Sedlock et al.[7] examined the accuracy (concurrent validity) of subject-palpated carotid and radial pulses compared to measures obtained with an ECG during exercise. Neither site proved to yield measures that were significantly different from those obtained from the gold standard.

Predictive
No data found.

Responsiveness
Not reported.

IMPORTANT REFERENCES ARE FOUND ON PAGE 199.

C.2. Blood Pressure

DESCRIPTION

A classically acknowledged vital sign, blood pressure is a measure of the pressure exerted within arterial walls during the two phases of the cardiac cycle, systole and diastole. It may be measured directly with an intra-arterial device or indirectly with an anaeroid sphygmomanometer and a stethoscope — the focus of this report. Indirect measures may underestimate the 'true' reading (taken directly) by 3-10 mmHg. A simple test, it was designed for screening, treatment planning, prediction and research. Physical therapists commonly use the measure for treatment planning and evaluation, especially as a response to physical exertion.

Population	Time to Complete	Cost	Training
Children and adult, normal or suspected or established cardiorespiratory problem.	One measure: less than 1 minute.	Anaeroid Sphygmomanometer $40-$90

mercury sphygmomanometer $65-$275 depending on the sophistication of the instrument. | Professional qualification. |

INSTRUCTIONS

There are a multitude of text references detailing the instructions for taking this measure and interpreting the pressures obtained. The most recent guidelines were published by the American Heart Association in 1988.

SCALING

Format

No active participation is required of the individual being assessed.

Subscales

Inherent.

Scoring

There are a wide variety of published reference values for both systolic and diastolic pressures. Age and sex are the main determinants of these normative ranges; however, many factors may influence any single measurement.

RELIABILITY

Internal consistency: Not reported.

Intrarater Reliability: Not reported.

Interrater Reliability

In Eilertsen and Humerfelt's classic study[1] nineteen specially trained nurses made measurements on 70,445 subjects using a conventional sphygmomanometer and a special apparatus designed to eliminate observer digit preference. They recorded diastolic pressures at the fourth and fifth Korotkoff sounds. Descriptive statistics and correlation coefficients were reported based on sex and age specific values. Consistent and substantial differences between readings were noted. In a study[2] to compare single and means of triplicate measures of blood pressure at two different visits in two positions (n = 40 hypertensive patients), the coefficient of variation of the single measures was 8.4%, while the coefficient of variation of the means of triplicate measures was 8.0%.

VALIDITY

Content (domain or face):

Not available.

Construct:

Not available.

Concurrent

Various studies[3-6] have compared direct and indirect measurement of arterial blood pressure and show: correlation coefficients, systolic (at rest) 0.89-0.95; diastolic (using the fourth Korotkoff sound) 0.83-0.88, and (using the fifth Korotkoff sound) 0.82-0.93.

During exercise, systolic pressure measured indirectly may be accurate and reliable, but not diastolic pressure.[3,4] Direct measures may yield smaller variations with increasing intensity of exercise.[6] Stolt et al.[7] compared direct intraarterial measures of blood pressure with a standard cuff and a new kind of cuff containing three rubber bags of different sizes, which automatically selects the appropriately sized bag in relation to arm circumference. Too small a cuff is known to render falsely high readings.[8-12]

In 48 individuals, the mean difference between the intraarterial and standard cuff blood pressures was 3+/-10 / -8+/-9 mmHg (systolic/diastolic), p. < 0.05/.001. With the new cuff, the mean difference was 5+/-9/-5+/-8 mmHg, p. < 0.001/.001. The calculated coefficients for each were all greater than 0.92. Values for sensitivity and specificity for systolic and diastolic pressures calculated for both cuffs showed no significant difference in specificity and sensitivity for systolic pressure. There was a significant difference (p. <0.005) between the specificity of the two devices when measuring diastolic blood pressure, but the new cuff proved more able to correctly identify 'normotensive' patients.

Predictive: Not reported.

Responsiveness: Not reported.

IMPORTANT REFERENCES ARE FOUND ON PAGE 199.

C.3.   Respiratory Rate

DESCRIPTION

One of the vital signs, respiratory rate is simply a measure of the number of breaths (respiratory cycles) per minute. It may be measured by a number of sophisticated laboratory technologies, but clinically is performed by inspection or palpation of the chest wall. A simple test, it was designed for screening, treatment planning, prediction and research. Physical therapists commonly use the measure for treatment planning and evaluation, especially as a response to physical exertion. The frequency of breathing is one of the determinants of ventilation, along with tidal volume. It is frequently used as an overall indicator of the status of the respiratory system.

Population	Time to Complete	Cost	Training
Children and adults, normal or with cardiorespiratory problems.	Cycles counted over 30 or 60 seconds.	None.	Professional qualification.

INSTRUCTIONS

There are a multitude of basic text references and guidelines available for the performance of the technique. Ranges of normal vary with age.

SCALING

Format
No active participation is required of the individual being assessed.

Subscales
None reported.

Scoring
Respiratory rate is recorded in breaths per minute.

RELIABILITY

Internal consistency

Not available.

Intrarater Reliability

Simoes et al.[1] measured respiratory rates in children by observation and using a pneumogram. Their aim was to determine the optimal counting interval (using two 30 sec and one 60 sec interval), to examine the effect of age and 'state' of the child on accuracy, to determine the natural variability in respiratory rate over a one hour period, and to calculate failure rates in obtaining a measure.

They concluded that counting for a 60-second interval or in 2 periods of 30 seconds was more accurate than counting for 30 seconds and doubling the rate. The variability in the measures was highest in children between 2-11 months, in those who were agitated, and in those who had an upper respiratory tract infection (as opposed to lower respiratory tract involvement or normals). Within one individual over the space of an hour, 50% of the 60 sec counts varied by up to 14 breaths/minute, and 75% by up to 21 breaths/minute. Failure rates fell somewhere between 10-16% and were greatest in infants less than 2 months of age and those who were agitated.

Similar kinds of investigations could not be found on adult subjects in the recent literature.

Interrater Reliability

Not available.

VALIDITY

Content (domain or face)

Not reported.

Construct

Not reported.

Concurrent

Not reported.

Predictive

Not reported.

Responsiveness.

Not reported.

IMPORTANT REFERENCES ARE FOUND ON PAGE 200.

C.4. Percussion

DESCRIPTION

The quality of sound elicited by tapping the chest wall in a systematic manner is used to evaluate the density of underlying lung tissue. It is most commonly performed by tapping the third digit of the non-dominant hand (the pleximeter, which rests on the chest wall) with the distal interphalangeal joint of the third finger of the dominant hand (the plexor), so called mediate percussion. This clinical examination technique is used most commonly by physical therapists for screening, treatment planning, evaluation and research.

Population	Time to Complete	Cost	Training
Children (not neonates) and adults, normal or with respiratory problems.	Less than 3 minutes.	None.	Professional qualification.

INSTRUCTIONS

There are a multitude of basic text references and guidelines available for the performance of the technique. Guidelines for nomenclature and interpretation of elicited sounds vary widely as well. Parrino[1] includes one of the most recent descriptions that is fairly universal.

SCALING

Format

No active participation is required of the individual being assessed.

Subscales

Not applicable.

Scoring

No scoring system is applied, only the assignment of 3 or 5 basic auditory findings which would indicate the presence of normal air filled lung, more air containing tissue, or less air containing tissue.

RELIABILITY

Internal consistency and Intrarater Reliability

Agreement

Original reports of the repeatability and observer agreement of respiratory signs, including percussion, were made by Smyllie et al.[2] and Godfrey et al.[3] Using the standard deviation agreement index (SDAI) and the experience agreement index (EAI), they concluded that observer agreement for percussion fell midway between maximum or complete agreement and chance agreement.

Spiteri et al.[4] reported that sets of 4 physicians were in agreement only 55% of the time when assessing the presence or absence of respiratory signs in clients with definitive diagnoses confirmed by other investigations such as chest radiography and pulmonary function tests. Percussion was among the three most reliably elicited signs (kappa = 0.52 and 0.50).

In comparing conventional mediate percussion with a new methodology described by Guarino,[5] Bourke et al.[6] determined the sensitivity, specificity, positive and negative predictive values and diagnostic accuracy of both techniques. Chest radiographs were used as the gold standard. For the conventional technique under examination in this report, sensitivity was calculated to be 15.4%, specificity was 97.3%, positive predictive value was 66.7%, negative predictive value was 76.6% and diagnostic accuracy was 76%. The prevalence of radiological abnormalities in the 100 lung fields (n = 50 clients) assessed was 26%.

VALIDITY

Content (domain or face)
Not available.

Construct
Not available.

Concurrent
See Bourke et al.[6] work as reported above.

Predictive
Not reported.

Responsiveness
The sensitivity of percussion, as reported by Bourke et al.[6] is low. All of the basic texts are in agreement that it is not sensitive at all to lesions 5 cm beyond the surface of the chest wall or to lesions less than 3 cm in diameter.[7]

IMPORTANT REFERENCES ARE FOUND ON PAGE 201.

C.5.   Auscultation of Lung Sounds

DESCRIPTION

Auscultation means the 'act of listening'. Though not a measurement, it should be considered in examination of outcome measures. It is the most universally taught technique of physical examination of the chest. Breath sounds from a stethoscope applied to the chest wall in a systematic fashion as the individual being examined creates an increased amount of turbulent airflow in the large airways are reported as normal (present), decreased, absent or abnormal (adventitious).

Population	Time to Complete	Cost	Training
Children and adults, normal or with cardiorespiratory problems.	3 minutes for a complete performance.	Basic stethoscope. $15 - $90	Professional qualification.

INSTRUCTIONS

There are a multitude of basic text references and guidelines available for the performance of the technique. Guidelines for nomenclature and interpretation of sounds vary widely as well. The most recent are based on international symposiums, such as that reported by Mikami et al.[1]

SCALING

Format

Under optimal circumstances, the individual breathes deeply through his/her mouth in an upright position during the assessment.

Subscales

None.

Scoring

No scoring system is applied, only the assignment of internationally agreed upon terminology to the presence of specific abnormal or adventitious sounds.

RELIABILITY

Agreement

Original reports of the repeatability and observer agreement of respiratory signs, including auscultation were made by Schilling and Hughes,[2] Smyllie et al.[3], Schneider and Anderson and Godfrey et al.[4] They basically concluded (using various statistics) that observer agreement for lung sounds fell midway between complete agreement and chance agreement.

More recently, Pasterkamp et al.[5] found considerable intra- and interobserver variability in the use of terms to describe adventitious sounds. While descriptive statistics only were reported, physiotherapists had the highest degree of agreement in terminology and this was thought to be due to their participation in regular inservices.

Spiteri et al.[6] reported that sets of 4 physicians were in agreement only 55% of the time when assessing the presence or absence of respiratory signs in clients with definitive diagnoses confirmed by other investigations such as chest radiography and pulmonary function tests. Kappa values for identification of wheezes (k=0.51), pleural rub (k=0.51), reduced breath sounds (k=0.41), crackles (k=0.41) and bronchial breathing (k=0.32) were reported. The mean pair agreement index indicated that this degree of agreement fell approximately midway between chance and total agreement.

Specific to physical therapists (in general practice as well as those 'specialized' in cardiorespirology), Aweida and Kelsey[7] and Brooks et al.,[8] used tape recorded lung sounds to assess the accuracy of sound identification (determined to be approximately 50% in both groups) and interrater reliability (reported as fair, kappa = 0.22 for 'generalists'; 0.26 for 'specialists').

VALIDITY

Content (domain or face)

Construct

Concurrent

Predictive

Responsiveness
Not reported.

IMPORTANT REFERENCES ARE FOUND ON PAGE 201.

C.6. Chronic Respiratory Disease Questionnaire (CRQ)

DESCRIPTION

The chronic respiratory disease questionnaire (CRQ) was developed by Gordon Guyatt et al.[1] for use as a clinical measure of quality of life of clients with chronic lung disease both in planning and evaluating therapeutic strategies, and for research. Its 4 dimensions include 20 questions (total) regarding: i)dyspnea, ii)fatigue, iii)emotional function and iv)mastery (the extent to which an individual feels in control or able to cope with illness).

Population	Time to Complete	Cost	Training
Adults with disability/handicap resulting from chronic lung disease.	Initial administration: 30 minutes max (average 15-25); follow up: 20 minutes max (average 10-15).	Kit $50.	The information with the kit is adequate. Professional qualification is required.

INSTRUCTIONS

The kit contains background information, explicitly written instructions (along with an audiotape) for administering the instrument, follow-up questionnaire, large print response cards, a response sheet, sample scores and their interpretation.

SCALING

Format

Questionnaire - self report.

Subscales

Not applicable.

Scoring

Each item has 7 response options (presented in Likert scale form), 7 being the best possible function and 1 the worst. The scores for each of the 4 dimensions are added together. Minimum and maximum scores for each dimension are delineated in the kit. Instructions for the determination of minimal clinically important change are clearly outlined.

RELIABILITY

Internal consistency and Intrarater Reliability

N/A

Interrater Reliability

Guyatt et al.[1] administered the instrument to 25 clients with stable chronic airflow limitation, 6 times at 2-week intervals. Calculated coefficients of variation for the four dimensions were as follows: 6% dyspnea; 9% fatigue and emotional function; 12% mastery.

VALIDITY

Content (domain or face)
Construct

Theoretically, since the questionnaire was formulated based on statements gathered in semi-structured interviews with clients, the responses should reflect their concerns, and therefore, their quality of life. As well, the scores appear to be stable in clients who are deemed to be stable, and improve when improvement is anticipated.

Concurrent

Guyatt et al.[1] compared measures of forced expiratory volume in the first second (FEV_1), slow vital capacity (SVC), 6-minute walk test, oxygen cost diagram, and global ratings of dyspnea, fatigue, etc., to related dimensions in the CRQ. The dyspnea dimension and 6-minute walk test had an r value of 0.46, clients' global rating of dyspnea and the dyspnea dimension, r = 0.37, clients' report of fatigue and the fatigue dimension, r = 0.42, clients' global rating of emotional function and the emotional dimension of the CRQ, r = 0.35. Later, Guyatt et al.[2] calculated simple and partial correlations of the Rand dyspnea questionnaire, the Rand physical and emotional function questionnaire, the oxygen cost diagram and the CRQ to FEV_1,[2] 6-minute walk test and visual analogue scale for dyspnea after the walk test. In each case, the CRQ was found to be the more valid (and sensitive) indicator of disability.

In an randomized control trial, Guyatt et al.[3] found that the validity of the CRQ might be improved if subjects were allowed to see their previous responses (i.e. an informed condition).

Predictive

Not available.

Responsiveness

Guyatt et al.[2] reported statistically significant changes in all 4 dimensions when tested before and 2-6 weeks after alterations of treatment and participation in an inpatient respiratory rehabilitation program. The CRQ was also compared concurrently before and after a respiratory rehabilitation program to the oxygen cost diagram, transition dyspnea index, Rand dyspnea questionnaire and emotional function questionnaire. The t values of the CRQ and the transition dyspnea index were similar, but the CRQ t values were consistently higher than the other measures, apparently confirming the CRQ's greater sensitivity to clinical change.

IMPORTANT REFERENCES ARE FOUND ON PAGE 202.

C.7. Visual Analogue Scale for DYSPNEA (VAS)

DESCRIPTION

There are a number of clinical rating scales which have been developed to quantify dyspnea, usually defined as the unpleasant sensation of laboured or difficult breathing, synonymous with the terms breathlessness or shortness of breath. Introduced by Aitken[1] the VAS is commonly represented as either a 100 mm or a 30 cm line, horizontal or vertical, with only two verbal expressions at the extreme ends: at one end, 'minimum shortness of breath' or 'not at all breathless' at the other, 'maximum breathlessness' or 'worst possible breathlessness'. Individuals choose a point on the line that best represents their current degree of breathlessness. It is a measure to be used serially with the aim of understanding one individual's perceived shortness of breath. Children must have fully developed communication skills. It is primarily used by physical therapists as a clinical measure for planning and evaluating treatment as well as for research.

Population	Time to Complete	Cost	Training
Pediatric (with fully developed communication skills) and adults, with cardio-respiratory problems.	Less than 1 min.	None.	Professional qualification.

INSTRUCTIONS

Variations in the scale's design and use exist in the literature. Mahler[2] describes it most currently and discusses guidelines for interpretation.

SCALING

Format

Self-report (the individual must be able to "partition a sensory continuum over a closed range"[3]).

Subscales

Not applicable.

Scoring

Score may be obtained by measuring the distance from minimum end of scale (far left or bottom, depending on the line's orientation) to the individual's chosen mark on the line (reported in cm or mm).

RELIABILITY

Internal consistency: Not applicable.

Intrarater Reliability: Not applicable.

Interrater Reliability: Not applicable.

Parallel-forms Reliability

See Gift[4] under **Concurrent Validity** (below).

Reproducibility

Muza[3] determined a coefficient of variation (between exercise tests on stable COPD clients) of $6 \pm 1\%$ (see below).

VALIDITY

Content (domain or face)

The face validity of a 100mm horizontal VAS was reportedly confirmed by Adams et al.[5] with 3 different groups of normal subjects chemically and physically challenged to experience breathlessness.

Construct

Using a contrasted groups approach (asthmatics and COPD clients representing acute and chronic dyspnea "experiences"), Gift[4] calculated t-test scores under conditions of severe and mild obstruction as defined by Peak Expiratory Flow Rate (PEFR). The t values of 12.35 (asthmatics) and 9.73 (COPD) at $p < 0.01$ demonstrated construct validity of the vertical VAS in both populations.

Concurrent

Muza[3] compared a 30 cm vertical VAS with the Borg scale of perceived exertion (both converted to Z scores): $r = 0.94$, $p < 0.01$. Six stable COPD clients performed 2 progressive incremental exercise tests on one day and a third test 10 days later. The VAS correlated highly to oxygen consumption ($r = 0.96$ +/- 0.01), as did the Borg scale ($r = 0.96$ +/- 0.02). The VAS was also highly correlated to ventilation ($r = 0.98$ +/- 0.01). This value is similar to that obtained by Adams et al.[5] in normal subjects tested repeatedly over 1 day and 1 week (r value fell to 0.64 at one year).

Gift[4] examined concurrent validity between horizontal and vertical VAS (actually, alternate forms of reliability). The former was considered to be the standard or criterion. She also used peak expiratory flow rate (PEFR) as a criterion against which the vertical VAS was compared. The r value for the vertical and horizontal VAS was 0.97, while the vertical scale and PEFR achieved an r value of -0.85. The vertical scale was judged preferable because of better client comprehension.

Predictive: Not available.

Responsiveness

Muza et al[3] and Wilson and Jones[6] suggest that the VAS is more sensitive to clinically important change than the Borg scale. Muza[3] found the former to possess twice the resolution of the latter. It may be, however, that this difference is due to the inherent differences in the physical dimensions of the two scales.

IMPORTANT REFERENCES ARE FOUND ON PAGE 202.

C.8.   Six-Minute Walking Test

DESCRIPTION

Cooper[1,2] developed the original 12-minute walking test as a field test for assessing maximal oxygen uptake in athletes. It was then modified for estimating the $VO_{2\,max}$ of disabled populations by McGavin et al.[3,4] The timing of the test was altered by Butland et al.[5] It may be performed on a treadmill or as a free walk over a pre-measured distance. Parameters measured during performance include heart rate, blood pressure, respiratory rate, oxygen saturation and degree of dyspnea or perceived exertion. While it is not reported in the literature, personal experience has proven that one test in its entirety, measuring all the suggested variables above (performed as a free walk), including baseline and resting/recovery measures, takes less than a half-hour. While investigating the effect of encouragement on 2 and 6-minute walking tests, Guyatt et al.[6] concluded that the 6-minute version was more responsive to change in client's status. Inconsistent administration of the test was felt to cause enough variation in distance walked to mask treatment effects. They also confirmed the existence of the training effect, which makes three performances of the test necessary for an accurate reflection of functional exercise capacity.

Population	Time to Complete	Cost	Training
Children or adults, particularly with cardiorespiratory problems.	Approximately 20-30 minutes.	None.	Professional qualification.

INSTRUCTIONS

Before 1984, the 12-minute test (and its subsequent modifications) was modelled after the descriptions provided by Cooper and McGavin. Guyatt et al.[6-8] addressed the lack of standardization of the performance of the test in the literature and the importance of administering the test in a consistent fashion (e.g. with or without encouragement). Cooper provided a table of predicted maximal oxygen consumption values on the basis of 12-minute performance (for normal subjects). The literature is consistent in its recommendation that the test be performed 3 times, with the distance covered in the third test being the most accurate reflection of the individual's performance.

SCALING

Format

   Task performance, specifically, walking.

Subscales

   Not applicable.

Scoring

   Individual performance is usually measured in distance covered in the six minute time interval. In the literature, this is reported in either meters or feet.

RELIABILITY

Internal consistency Intrarater Reliability
Interrater Reliability

McGavin's[4] test of 62 clients with obstructive lung disease and acute pulmonary infiltrates revealed test-retest r values within one individual (tested twice with a 20 minute interval) to be 0.97 (p <0.001), but the group mean of the second test was significantly greater. Tests of 13 chronic bronchitic clients 6 times at 2-3 week intervals confirmed there was a significant difference between the first three performances of the test. The coefficient of variation for all subjects over all the tests was ±8.2%. This was reduced to ±4.2% if the first two tests were discarded.[9]

VALIDITY

Content (domain or face)
Construct

Based on Cooper's work, the distance covered by normal individuals in the 12-minute walk-run test was highly correlated with the $VO_{2\ max}$ determined in the laboratory (r = 0.897). In subsequent investigations, the distance covered does appear to improve when improvements are anticipated in client status.

Concurrent

Conflicting reports exist on the test's correlation with pulmonary function tests.[3,4,9-13] Some believe performance is mostly due to pathophysiological factors, while others believe psychological and motivational factors predominate. McGavin et al.[3] found r values of 0.52 and 0.53 between the 12 minute walking distance (in chronic bronchitic clients) and VO_2 and V_E values determined with progressive bicycle ergometry testing.

Significant correlations have been reported between the 6 and 12-minute walking tests and tests such as the oxygen cost diagram (r = 0.68, p <0.001, r = 0.37, p = 0.01) structured questionnaires regarding symptomology, Rand Instrument (r = 0.31; r = 0.589), the Baseline Dyspnea Index (r = 0.59), Specific Activity Scale (r = 0.473) and the Chronic Respiratory Disease Questionnaire (r = 0.52, p = 0.01).[8,10,13]

Some studies examined the correlation between walking tests and other forms of exercise testing. Swinburn et al.[16] compared 12-minute walking test results to cycle ergometry and a step test and found no correlations with spirometric measures. All showed improvement with practice (the 12-minute test showing the least degree of variability). Guyatt et al.[8] calculated an r value of 0.579 between the 6-minute walking test and cycle ergometry (performed by 43 clients with chronic heart failure and chronic lung disease). The latter test did not correlate with other functional measures of performance.

Beaumont et al.[14] and Swerts et al.[15] compared the 12-minute walking test performed on a 'self-paced' treadmill and as a free walk in a corridor, by 6 severely breathless clients. Beaumont et al. did not find a significant difference (p >0.1) in distance covered by the 2 methods, and generally, favoured the use of the treadmill as it enabled monitoring of heart rate with an electrocardiogram and oxygen saturation with an ear oximeter.[14] Severely involved COPD clients performed better in the corridor, although heart rate and dyspnea measures were comparable, recommending the free walk.

IMPORTANT REFERENCES ARE FOUND ON PAGE 203.

C.9. Self-Paced Walking Test to predict $V0_2$ max

DESCRIPTION

Aerobic capacity is an important measure of physical capacity.[1] Direct measures of $V0_2$ are expensive and impractical in the clinical setting. Various forms of sub-maximal tests for predicting $V0_2$ max are in use. One such test is the use of self-paced walking. Here again, there are a variety of protocols in use. There has been extensive work done on the effects of aging on walking pace and age/gender specific normative data has been collected. The test was developed as a measure of cardiovascular fitness and is used as a performance index, as the test is sensitive to age differences. The self-paced walking test is starting to be used as a predictor of $V0_2$ max in the back injured population. To date no literature has been found on its use specifically in back injured individuals. One of the protocols used is described by Bassey[2] and is summarized below.

Population	Time to Complete	Cost	Training
Normal individuals, chronic respiratory disease, back disabilities.	Less than 10 minutes.	Minimum equipment: stop watch, heart rate monitor, pylons to mark the course.	None required.

INSTRUCTIONS

The subject is asked to walk a course of 128 meters, 3 times at graded paces: "slow", "normal pace, neither fast nor slow" and "rather fast without over exerting yourself". The heart rate, time to complete the distance and the number of strides are recorded.

SCALING

Format

Task performance.

Subscales

None.

Scoring

The velocity is calculated in m/sec. The 0_2 cost ($V0_2$) can be extrapolated from aerobic demand curves.[3] The estimated $V0_2$ max can then be extrapolated using the $V0_2$ and the heart rate.[1]

Internal consistency

The variation in the number of strides and the time to complete each lap was plus or minus 3-6%.[2,3]

Test-retest Reliability

A variability of 4.7 - 11% was found in the test-retest situation. The 11% variability was found at the slow walking speeds.[2,3]

Interrater Reliability

Not reported.

VALIDITY

Content (domain or face)

Content validity is only fair as it tests not only the cardiorespiratory transport system but is heavily influenced by the mechanics of walking and limitations due to pain and mood.

Construct

Not available.

Concurrent

In young and elderly males, there was moderate correlation found between O_2 uptake tests on the bicycle ergometer and the self-paced walking ($r = 0.79$ at the $p < 0.001$ level).[2]

Predictive

Not available.

IMPORTANT REFERENCES ARE FOUND ON PAGE 204.

C.10. VITAL CAPACITY (Slow VC or Forced VC)

DESCRIPTION

In terms of static lung volumes, vital capacity represents the combination of inspiratory reserve volume, tidal volume and expiratory reserve volume (or total lung capacity minus residual volume), i.e. the volume of air moved from a point of maximal inspiration to maximal expiration as a slow expiratory manoeuvre (SVC) or a forced expiratory manoeuvre (FVC). It was designed to assist in the classification of non-obstructive respiratory impairments, determine the severity of a defect and so provide a method of tracking the course of a disease process, as well as selecting appropriate therapeutic management strategies. It is commonly used and interpreted in conjunction with other pulmonary function tests. Guidelines for measurement and interpretation are provided by the American Thoracic Society (ATS).[1,2] Physical therapists use this measure most to assess effects of surgery on the respiratory system and management strategies aimed at volume recovery and cough effectiveness. Another application is monitoring clients with neuromuscular disease (and so, respiratory impairment) and/or those being weaned from mechanical ventilation. Required are a vital capacity single gauge measurement device (spirometer); there are also battery operated, hand held portable spirometers which measure forced vital capacity as well as forced expiratory volume in the first second (FEV_1) and peak expiratory flow rate (PEFR).

Population	Time to Complete	Cost	Training
Age 8 years and up and adults, with suspected or established respiratory problems.	Depends on repetitions needed to satisfy the ATS standards.	Approximately $300-$800. Portable device: $2500-$3000. Nose clips: $2 each.	Minimal specific tech. instruction (guidelines, ref. values, etc.) beyond professional qualification.

INSTRUCTIONS
A multitude of standard texts and instructional manuals detail this simple manoeuvre.

SCALING

Format: Individual performance of prescribed manoeuvre.

Subscales: Not applicable.

Scoring

There are a wide variety of published reference values, and, therefore, interpretations of data. The 1991 document from the ATS[2] has attempted to clarify the issues surrounding the selection of reference values and interpretive strategies. Age, sex, height and ethnicity appear to be the most influential factors in the determination of normal ranges of vital capacity measures. It should be noted that the use of a fixed percent of predicted values to determine "normality" is discouraged.

RELIABILITY

Agreement

FVC is among the most reliable of the standard spirometric measures. Biologic within subject variability (calculated coefficients of variation in normals) ranges from 1.96 to 4.5%, over periods of one day, several weeks and several months (test-retest reliability). Coefficients of variation have been calculated on groups of clients with known respiratory diagnoses.[3-5] In each case, the variability was greater with pathology.

Although not calculated, **test specificity** is described as being excellent,[8] primarily because normal reference values vary to such a great degree. Test sensitivity is described as being poor, particularly where slight to moderate abnormalities are involved.[8-10]

VALIDITY

Content (domain or face)

Not available.

Construct

FVC is thought to reflect only the function of large airways, not peripheral ones of less than 2 mm diameter.[3,4,6,7]

Concurrent

While no calculated statistics were found, the vital capacity measurement is seldom performed in isolation. Diagnostic validity is believed to increase if a battery of pulmonary function tests is performed.

Predictive

Not available.

Responsiveness

Arbitrarily set limits for clinically significant change have been used widely in the past. Nickerson and associates[5] recommended an equation to calculate the specific percent change within subjects required for significance. This kind of simple calculation would certainly improve the accuracy of data interpretation.

IMPORTANT REFERENCES ARE FOUND ON PAGE 205.

C.11. PEAK EXPIRATORY FLOW RATE (PEFR)

DESCRIPTION

Peak expiratory flow rate is one of a group of forced expiratory flow measures taken at specific lung volumes — in this case, at total lung capacity or at the point of maximal inspiration. These measures, as a group, are thought to be indicative of small airway function, although there remains considerable debate about this in the literature. There are a variety of peak flow meters available. There are also battery operated, hand held portable spirometers which measure forced vital capacity (FVC), forced expiratory volume in the first second (FEV_1) as well as PEFR. Guidelines for measurement and interpretation are provided by the American Thoracic Society (ATS).[1,2] The text by Clausen is also helpful.[3]

Population	Time to Complete	Cost	Training
Children (8 years and up) and adults; normal or with suspected or established respiratory problems particularly airway hyperreactivity.	Depends on the repetitions to satisfy ATS standards. Instructions with the various devices marketed. Usually best recording of three attempts.	Ranging in price from $35-$60 The portable devices cost $2500-$3000 Nose clips: $2 each.	Minimal specific techn. instruction (guidelines, ref. values, etc.) beyond professional qualification.

INSTRUCTIONS

A multitude of standard texts and instructional manuals detail this simple manoeuvre.

SCALING

Format
Individual performance of prescribed manoeuvre.

Subscales
Not applicable.

Scoring
There are several published reference values and guidelines regarding interpretation. Age, sex and height are the most influential factors. The PEFR is an effort dependent measure. A percent fall from baseline during exercise, calculated by Clausen[3] may be appropriate for the determination of exercise induced asthma. Reference tables for client use are usually represented as lower limits of normality.

RELIABILITY

Internal consistency

Not applicable.

Intrarater Reliability

Not applicable.

Interrater Reliability

Not applicable.

Agreement

The biologic within-subject variability is greater in PEFR measures than for FVC. Circadian rhythms in healthy individuals have a peak-to-trough amplitude of approximately 8%.[4] This diurnal variation is known to be even greater in clients with chronic obstructive lung disease, including asthma.[5-9]

VALIDITY

Content (domain or face)

Not reported.

Construct

In total, all of the measures from the maximum expiratory flow rate curves are thought to best represent changes in small airways (Cosio et al;[10] Thurlbeck;[11] Tashkin et al.[8])

Concurrent

Not reported.

Predictive

Not reported.

Responsiveness

Arbitrarily set limits for clinically significant change have been used widely in the past. Percent changes of 10%, 15% and 20% have been used for normals. Larger percent changes must be used to detect clinically significant change where lung pathology is involved.

IMPORTANT REFERENCES ARE FOUND ON PAGE 206.

C.12. Maximum Inspiratory & Expiratory Pressures (MIP/MEP or MIF/MEF or PImax/PEmax)

DESCRIPTION

Rohrer[1] and Rahn[2] were first to point out in the literature that the pressure that a muscle develops is an index of its force. These maximal inspiratory and maximal expiratory manoeuvres were developed as measures of inspiratory and expiratory muscle strength respectively. The individual must create a maximum inspiratory or expiratory effort (at specific lung volumes) against an occluded airway. These tests were designed for clinical practice, screening, treatment planning and evaluation and research. Physical therapists use them mostly to evaluate respiratory muscle strength in clients undergoing ventilatory muscle training programs (breathing spontaneously or mechanically ventilated/weaning).

Population	Time to Complete	Cost	Training
Children and adults who are able to cooperate and comprehend.	Depends on the number performed. Most often 3 are obtained with 5% spread.	Simple hand-held pressure manometer with a Y valve and mouthpiece $80-$100 Nose clips: $2 each	Minimal specific tech. instruction and professional qualification.

INSTRUCTIONS

Various studies have employed a number of testing techniques, equipment and interpretive guidelines. Clausen's text[3] may be helpful in the clarity of its protocol, although there is still controversy regarding the measurement of MIP from residual volume or functional residual capacity. The methods of Black and Hyatt[4] for spontaneously breathing individuals and Marini et al.[5] for mechanically ventilated clients are most often cited. Rubenstein et al.[6] found that the various methods used to assess MEP's account for the large range of normal values existing in the literature.

SCALING

Format

Individual performance of prescribed manoeuvre.

Subscales

Not applicable.

Scoring

Interpretation of data is based on reference norms, which are variable as noted previously. Smyth et al.[7] and Wilson et al.[8] cautioned against using normal values from the existing literature.

RELIABILITY

Internal consistency

Not applicable.

Intrarater Reliability

Not applicable.

Interrater Reliability

Not applicable.

Agreement

Intrasubject variability, performing multiple trials (and recording maximum values obtained) in mechanically ventilated clients was found to be 18% (coefficient of variation) by Marini et al.[5] Rubenstein et al.[6] found within-subject coefficient of variation of 5-6% with scuba mouthpieces, 9-13% with tube technique (for MEP determination). Between-subject coefficients of variation were similar for men and women regardless of technique.

VALIDITY

Content (domain or face)

Not available.

Construct

There is agreement in the literature that the relationship between MIP and MEP generated at different lung volumes is a measure of the force-length properties of respiratory muscles.[9]

Concurrent

Rubenstein et al.[6] reported a close relationship between esophageal pressure (Pes) and mouth pressure (Pm), measured at FRC ($r = 0.98$, $p < 0.001$), indicating the validity of measuring mouth pressures to represent intrapulmonary pressure.

There continues to be conflicting data in the literature about MIP's relationship to vital capacity.

Predictive

Not available.

Responsiveness

Not available.

IMPORTANT REFERENCES ARE FOUND ON PAGE 207.

C.13. Oxygen Saturation

DESCRIPTION

Oxygen saturation represents the percent saturation of available blood hemoglobin. Approximately 19.7/20 ml of oxygen in 100 ml blood is carried bound to hemoglobin. The relationship between percent saturation and the partial pressure of oxygen in arterial blood (PaO_2) is described by the oxyhemoglobin dissociation curve. Values may be obtained in various ways: from a nomogram based on the oxyhemoglobin dissociation curve, measured by an oximeter directly with an arterial blood gas sample or from an ear oximeter, a pulse oximeter, or a transcutaneous oxygen monitoring system. The latter 3 non-invasive innovations provide continuous data. The pulse oximeter (SpO_2), providing the fastest growing and most commonly utilized methodology, represents a combination of oximetry and plethysmographic technologies for screening, treatment planning and evaluation and research. Physical therapists use it often to monitor O_2 prescription and therapeutic strategies (in acutely ill or stable clients), including response to exercise.

Population	Time to Complete	Cost	Training
Children and adults with suspected or established cardiorespiratory problems.	Variable Pulse oximeter's continuous read-out, gives information instantaneously.	Available devices: $2000 to $6000	Minimal specific technical instruction (on the use of the device) beyond the professional qualification.

INSTRUCTIONS

Instructions on the use of a pulse oximeter are somewhat design/model specific.

SCALING

Format

No active participation is required of the individual being assessed.

Subscales

Not applicable.

Scoring

Hypoxia is defined as a PaO < 60mm Hg or a SaO < 90% (Ontario Ministry of Health).

RELIABILITY

Internal consistency

Intrarater Reliability

Interrater Reliability

Agreement

Reliability in this context relates to the technology's ability to perform consistently. Clayton et al.[2] evaluated 20 different models of pulse oximeters in clients with poor perfusion, and found only 2 capable of clinically acceptable accuracy. Similar concerns have been expressed about the pulse oximeter's ability to perform during severe exercise or under other conditions of physiological extremes.[3,4]

VALIDITY

Content (domain or face)

Construct

Concurrent

Pulse oximetry has acceptable accuracy in the 70-100% range, based on a comparison of SpO_2 to SaO_2 from a co-oximeter that analyzed arterial blood gas samples (r = 0.98).[5] Work by Taylor and Whotwam[4] confirmed similar r values with five different models of pulse oximeters, but noted consistent underestimation of the actual SaO_2.

Ries[6] and Severinghaus[7] reported accuracy of +/- 3-5% at saturations above 70% (95% confidence intervals). The mean difference between the values obtained by the pulse oximeter and the gold standard (SaO_2 analyzed from an arterial blood gas sample) is the bias and the standard deviation of the differences is precision. Nickerson et al.[8] found bias in the measurement to be 1-2%, while precision was 2-4% (in saturations above 80%). This was felt to be acceptable performance for clinical decision making.

A review of studies[3] revealed precision values within +/- 2-3% when SaO_2 is greater than 90%; precision would be +/- 4-6% if a 95% confidence interval is required. The report recommends that a lower limit of acceptability of SpO_2 be 92% in white clients and 95% in black clients.

Predictive

Not reported.

Responsiveness

The pulse oximeter is insensitive in clients with relatively high levels of oxygenation, but increasingly sensitive with greater degrees of hypoxia.[9]

A change of 1% (above 90%) and 2% (below 90%) would represent clinically significant change in normal individuals.[6]

IMPORTANT REFERENCES ARE FOUND ON PAGE 208.

D.1. Alberta Infant Motor Scale (AIMS)

DESCRIPTION

The AIMS is an observational measure used to identify infants whose motor performance is delayed or aberrant relative to a normative group.[1,2] It may be used to provide information to the clinician and to parents about the motor activities the child has mastered, those currently developing, and those not yet in the infant's repertoire. It was designed to evaluate the efficacy of rehabilitation programs for infants with motor dysfunction and to measure small change in motor performance. It can also be used as a research tool to assess the efficacy of rehabilitation programs. The AIMS analyzes the components used to achieve motor milestones. It evaluates the sequential development of postural control relative to four postural positions: supine, prone, sitting and standing. It observes three aspects of motor performance (weight bearing, posture and antigravity movements). The AIMS can also be used as a screening tool.

Population	Time to Complete	Cost	Training
Infants at risk of developing motor problems, from term through the age of independent walking.	15 min.	Requires minimal space and little special equipment.	None required.

INSTRUCTIONS

Each item consists of an artist's drawing of an infant in a particular position accompanied by a detailed description of the key descriptors that must be observed for the infant to pass the item.

SCALING

Format

Observation.

Subscales

The scale consists of 58 items divided into 4 positions:

Prone (21)
Supine (9)
Sitting (12)
Standing (16)

Scoring

Each item is scored on a nominal scale: Pass/Fail.

RELIABILITY

Internal consistency

Not reported.

Intrarater Reliability

Normal infants, 221 stratified by age from birth to 18 months of age were scored twice within 7 days. When the same rater was used (N=95), the correlation was high (.996). When different raters were used (N=138), the correlation was also high (0.993).[1]

Interrater Reliability

Those same infants, from birth to 18 months of age, were tested by 2 independent raters at the same testing period. The correlation between their scores was very high (0.998).[1]

VALIDITY

Content (domain or face)

Eighty-four items were generated based upon descriptions of early motor performance. They were separated into the four positions in which the infants are to be assessed: prone, supine, sitting, and standing. Albertan pediatric physical therapists as well as 291 members of the Pediatric Physical Therapy Division of the Canadian Physiotherapy Association were asked to rate the items as to their importance to motor development, and to sort the items as to their typical order of emergence and the age range within which each item should emerge.

A panel of 6 international experts in infant motor development discussed the items. Several revisions were made resulting in a total of 59 items. Ninety-seven infants, aged 0-18 months of age, were evaluated as part of a feasibility pretest.

Construct

Multidimensional scaling revealed that the data fit well into a one dimension – motor maturity index.
(Stress = .04; R^2 = .995)

The items formed an almost perfect Guttman scale. The total score correlated well with age in days (.95).

Concurrent

The Bayley Psychomotor Development Scale and the Peabody Developmental Motor Scales were administered to 12 infants from 0-13 months at the same time as the AIMS. The correlation between the AIMS and both the Bayley (.98) and the Peabody (.97) were excellent.

Predictive

Not reported.

Discriminative

Eighteen infants with diagnoses of abnormal motor development and 44 infants at risk for motor disorders were assessed. The results were compared with the tentative norms derived from the normal sample. Of the 18 children with abnormalities, 16 were considered abnormal on the AIMS (< 2 SD from the mean). Of the 44 at-risk children, 10 were considered suspicious and 3 abnormal.[2]

IMPORTANT REFERENCES ARE FOUND ON PAGE 208.

D.2. Bayley Scales of Infant Development (Psychomotor Scale)

DESCRIPTION

The Bayley[1] provides a comprehensive assessment of the motor and mental development of infants. It may be used clinically and for research.

Population	Time to Complete	Cost	Training
Children: birth – 36 months.	45 minutes to administer both the Psychomotor Developmental Index and the Mental Developmental Index.	Test kit required.	None required. Examiners should be familiar with the administration and scoring procedures of the Bayley.

INSTRUCTIONS

The detailed manual provides the directions for administering each item and the criteria for scoring.

SCALING

Format

Task performance.

Subscales

Consists of scales:
1. Mental scale
2. Psychomotor scale (head control, prone, supine, rolling, sit, stand, walk, balance, jump, line walk, grasp, manipulation).

Scoring

Scoring is based on a 2-point scale: Pass/Fail.

Performance is tested from the individual child's basal level to ceiling level. The raw score is converted to a developmental quotient. Age equivalent scores are also available. The Bayley Scales were standardized on 1,262 children ranging in age from 2 - 30 months, using standardized equipment and procedures.

RELIABILITY

Internal consistency

One thousand, nine hundred and thirty-five children aged 1-15 months were evaluated on the psychomotor index. Correlations between the items ranged from moderate to high (0.63 to 0.93).[2]

Intrarater Reliability

The children were evaluated twice within a one month interval. The correlations between the two tests ranged from low to high (.53 to .91).[2]

Interrater Reliability

One tester and one observer rated 90 children at 8 months of age. The correlations between the two sets of psychomotor scores were high (0.88 - 0.99).

VALIDITY

Content (domain or face)

Not reported.

Construct

The relationship between scores at 4, 8, 12 and 24 months of age was assessed. The correlation between Bayley scores at different ages ranged from poor to good (.52 - .84), with correlations generally better for the earliest years.[3] Sixty children were evaluated at a mean age of 4.3 months to determine the degree to which the items follow a normal developmental sequence. Correlations were high (0.89 - 0.84).[3]

Concurrent

Several studies have examined the concurrent validity of the Bayley using the Peabody Motor Scales with varying results. At 4 months the correlations were found to be either poor (.13) or good (0.67 - 0.83). At 12, 15, and 18 months the correlations for the gross motor scale were good (0.78 - 0.96) but poor for the fine motor scale (0.20 - 0.57).[4]

Predictive

A retrospective study of 70 children showed that 4, 12 and 24 month Bayley scores were poorly correlated to later cognitive performance.[5]

Eight month Bayley scores correlated poorly with 48 month Standford-Binet (.13-.15) and Graham-Ernhart Block Test (0.12-.014) scores.[6] Early psychomotor scores correlated poorly with language comprehension and expression scores at 2 years (0.337 - 0.55).

The Bayley scores can predict a 3-8 year diagnosis of cerebral palsy or neurological normality with a sensitivity of 94.9%,[7] and can predict the results of a 1 and 7 year neurological examination with a sensitivity of 59%.[8] Psychomotor tests performed on high-risk infants at 4 months adjusted age correlated poorly with WPPSI (0.05-0.13) and Peabody scores (0.004-0.13) at 4 1/2 years .

IMPORTANT REFERENCES ARE FOUND ON PAGE 209.

D.3. Peabody Developmental Motor Scale

DESCRIPTION

The Peabody was developed to identify children whose gross motor and fine motor skills are delayed or aberrant relative to a normative group.[1-11] This scale can also be used to design therapeutic interventions through the use of activity cards linked to the assessment items . The Peabody is designed to be used in clinical practice for screening, evaluation and program planning. It may also be used in research.

Population	Time to Complete	Cost	Training
Children 0-83 months with a spectrum of motor impairment from none or minimal to severe.	40-60 minutes. The test can be administered in groups of children 4 year old and above.	$135 U.S. (1984) for test kit, including manual and activity cards.	None required.

INSTRUCTIONS

The manual provides details on the materials required, the directions for administering each item, the criteria for scoring and suggestions for modifying the assessment procedure for children whose handicap precludes testing with standard version.

SCALING

Format

Task performance.

Subscales

The assessment consists of 2 scales:
The Gross Motor subscale (170 items divided into 17 age levels) covers 5 domains: reflexes; balance; non-locomotor mobility; locomotion; and ability to catch and throw.
The Fine Motor subscale (112 items divided into 6 age levels) covers 4 domains: grasping; hand use; eye-hand co-ordination; and manual dexterity.

Scoring

Each item has a criterion performance level specifying the number of trials permitted and the amount time allotted for completion. Scoring is on a 3-point ordinal scale:

> 0-unsuccessful;
> 1-clear resemblance to criterion, but criterion not fully met; or
> 2-successful performance.

A raw score is obtained for each specific domain and for each subscale. Scores are converted to an age equivalent, a developmental motor quotient, a percentile ranking, and a standardized score (Z or t). The raw score can be converted into a scaled score (an equal interval scale independent of age.) This is useful for detecting small changes in motor development in handicapped children.
Norms for various subgroups of children based on age, sex, race and geographical region were generated using serial evaluations of 617 children by multiple testers. The mean motor quotient of the normative sample at each age level is 100 (SD=15).

RELIABILITY

Internal consistency

The standard error (SE): gross motor subscale 1.10 - 5.39; fine motor 0.7 - 2.6.[1]

Intrarater Reliability

Thirty-eight children were tested twice in one week. The 2 tests showed correlations. For gross motor subscale the correlations between the 2 tests was 0.90; for the fine motor subscale the test-retest reliability was 0.95.[1]

Interrater Reliability

The same 30 children were also evaluated simultaneously by 2 independent evaluators. Their correlation on the gross motor subscale was 0.97 and 0.94 on the fine motor subscale. When 16 developmentally delayed and 16 normal children (all 4 - 5 years) were evaluated simultaneously by two independent raters, the intraclass correlation coefficient (ICC) was 0.76 for the normal group and 0.96 for the delayed group. Kappa statistics for individual items ranged from -0.09 to 0.92, with 30% of the items receiving less than 80% agreement.[2]

VALIDITY

Content (domain or face)

Items were based on established research on motor development and validated motor scales, and their order adheres to Harrow's hierarchical sequence of motor development.[1]

Construct

Significant incremental increase in scores was observed at each age level except that corresponding to 54 to 59 months. This age level did not differ significantly from the preceding age level.

Concurrent

Except at age level 0 to 5 months, scores on the items discriminated between 104 children with impaired motor development and a normative group.[1] When 23 full-term infants and 21 low risk pre-term infants were evaluated at 12, 15 and 18 months of (adjusted) age, the Gross Motor subscale correlated well with the Bayley Motor Scale (0.63-0.93); but the Fine Motor did not (0.17-0.23). Individual domains showed low to moderate correlations (0.36-.80).[7]

Predictive

When evaluated at 12, 15, and 18 months of (adjusted) age, 23 full-term and 21 pre-term infants showed the following correlations: 12 vs 18 months .25-.75; 12 vs 15 months .25-.85; and 15 vs 18 months .35-.72.[7]

Responsiveness

A clinical trial of 45 developmentally disabled children (aged 3 to 15 years) tested effectiveness of developmental therapy at two different intensities. The Peabody differentiated the treatment groups from the controls.[3] Similarly, the effectiveness of a program of controlled vestibular stimulation evaluated using the Peabody Motor Scales showed significant gains.[5] In 10 infants with Down's Syndrome (aged 6 to 42 weeks), evaluated twice over 6 weeks, provided no significant change (t=2.23 p >.05), in Peabody was observed. However, a significant difference using the Movement Assessment of Infants (MAI) was observed.[4]

IMPORTANT REFERENCES ARE FOUND ON PAGE 210.

D.4. Test of Motor and Neurological Functions (TMNF)

DESCRIPTION

The TMNF was designed to examine quality of movement among infants who demonstrate suspect or abnormal motor and neurological findings.[1-3] It is suggested that the Motor Scale or the Bayley Scales of Infant Development be used in conjunction with the TMNF to code for qualitative movement findings during functional motor skills. Very few infants in the 10 to 12 months age range were used for the validation study. Therefore, caution should be used when interpreting results of testing performed on children in this age range. Designed for use by pediatricians, occupational and physical therapists and others with training and background in interpreting motor and neurological functions in high-risk infants.

Population	Time to Complete	Cost	Training
Infants with suspect or abnormal motor and neurological function, from 3-12 months of age.	Less than 1/2 hour.	Requires a mat and the items required to administer the Bayley Scales of Infant Development.	Approximately 2 hours of training is needed for orientation to the testing procedure.

INSTRUCTIONS

A standardized procedure for item administration and detailed criteria for scoring each item on the test are provided.

SCALING

Format

Task Performance.

Subscales

The assessment consists of 31 items divided into 3 subscales:
1. muscle tone (7 items)
2. primitive reflexes (4 items)
3. automatic and equilibrium reactions (13 items)

The following qualitative movements are rated: components of head and neck posture, trunk posture, shoulder girdle, pelvis, transitional movements, upper and lower extremities, and hand use.

Scoring

Muscle tone - low scores indicate low tone, middle scores normal tone, and high scores indicate high tone.

Primitive reflexes - exaggerated to no response implying that the reflex is fully integrated.

Automatic and equilibrium reactions - absent to fully developed.

To calculate an index for each of the subtests, the item scores for the subtest cluster are summed. The presence or absence of each item on the qualitative movement section is recorded.

RELIABILITY

Internal consistency

Not reported.

Intrarater Reliability

Not reported.

Interrater Reliability

A group of 10 normal full-term and 13 high risk infants were evaluated. Two observers (OT and PT) simultaneously scored the same set of responses. The ICC for the subtests were high (0.93 - 0.97).[3]

VALIDITY

Content (domain or face)

Not reported.

Construct

Construct validity was evaluated by examining the various parts of the test for their relationship to each other. Correlations between the subtests were low (.11 - .56), indicating that each subtest is measuring distinctly different neurological functions.[3]

Concurrent

Not reported.

Predictive

Not reported.

Responsiveness

Not reported.

IMPORTANT REFERENCES ARE FOUND ON PAGE 211.

D.5. Test of Motor Impairment

DESCRIPTION

The Test of Motor Impairment was designed to measure the degree of gross motor and fine motor impairment. It can be used in clinical practice.[1]

Population	Time to Complete	Cost	Training
All children with IQ > 50, aged 5 to 14 years.	Approximately 20 minutes.	Minimal.	None Required.

INSTRUCTIONS

The equipment, starting position, general description of each task, and the criteria for pass or fail are included in the manual.[1] Modifications may be made to accommodate individual children's special needs.

SCALING

Format

Task Performance.

Subscales

The test is divided into 5 subscales:
1. Control and balance of the body while immobile
2. Control and coordination of the upper limbs
3. Control and coordination of the body while in motion
4. Manual dexterity with the emphasis on speed
5. Tasks which emphasize simultaneous movement and precision

Scoring

The test is scored on a 3-point ordinal scale. The total score represents the degree of impairment:
0 - Well-coordinated child
1 - Unilateral failure
2 - Failed item
10 - Total failure at an age level

RELIABILITY

Internal consistency

Not reported.

Test-retest Reliability

Two different testers assessed 24 children within a two day interval. Correlations were high, ranging from 0.79 - 1.00.

Interrater Reliability

Not reported.

VALIDITY

Content (domain or face)

Many of the items were selected based on the items on the Oseretsky Test of Motor Ability.

Construct

The degree of specificity between the 5 subscales was examined using a sample of 854 children. The scores in each subscale were correlated with the remaining 4 subscales. Correlations ranged from 0.15 - 0.38 (p <.005 to p =.05).[1]

Concurrent

Seven hundred and thirteen children were tested to determine the relationship of the test scores to social adjustment using the Bristol Social Adjustment Guides. The percentage of maladjustment among motor impaired children is 20.5% and among well coordinated children 5.8%.

Predictive

Not reported.

Responsiveness

Not reported.

IMPORTANT REFERENCES ARE FOUND ON PAGE 211.

D.6. Posture and Fine Motor Assessment of Infants (PFMAI)

DESCRIPTION

The PFMAI was developed to measure small changes in motor function of infants, particularly changes in qualitative motor behavior. The essential components of motor skills are evaluated according to a developmental scale. The PFMAI is used clinically to evaluate motor dysfunction and to develop therapeutic interventions for young infants.[1]

Population	Time to Complete	Cost	Training
All infants aged 2 to 6 months.	45 minutes.	None.	Not reported.

INSTRUCTIONS
Not reported.

SCALING

Format

Caregiver report.

Subscales

The test consists of 2 subscales.

Posture:
- Co-contraction of the muscle groups around the body's axis
- Automatic righting reactions
- Stability in antigravity positions
- Isolated movements of the neck and trunk
- Ability to sustain movement against gravity while in prone and supine

Fine Motor:
- Control of reach, grasp and manipulation of objects
- Approach to object
- Accuracy of grasp
- Maintenance of grasp
- Grasp pattern
- Finger and thumb movement
- Developmental level of manipulation

Scoring

Each item is scored on a 4-point ordinal scale. The child's best response is recorded.

RELIABILITY

Internal consistency

Not reported.

Test-retest Reliability

Thirty-three infants with a mean age of 4.3 months were tested twice within 2 days. The agreement between the two subscales of the PFMAI and the total score ranged from moderate to high (ICC: 0.85 - 0.94). The item-specific agreement ranged from low to high (ICC and weighted Kappa: 0.21 - 0.91) with the item testing the time the child is able to hold legs in space demonstrating the lowest reliability.[2]

Interrater Reliability

Forty infants with a mean age of 4.2 months were rated by 4 graduate students and the principal investigator. The agreement for the individual items was excellent (ICC: 0.91 - 1.0).[2]

VALIDITY

Content (domain or face)

Not reported.

Construct

Scores for 60 infants were correlated with chronological age to determine degree to which the items follow a normal developmental sequence. The correlations reported were excellent (0.89 - 0.94).[2]

Concurrent

Thirty-two infants with a mean age of 4.4 months were tested on the PFMAI and the Peabody Scales of Infant Development within a 4-day period. The correlation between the Peabody Gross Motor Scale and the PFMAI posture scale was good (0.83), and the correlation between the Peabody Fine Motor Scale and the PFMAI Fine Motor Scale was moderate (0.68).[2]

Predictive

Not reported.

Responsiveness

Not reported.

IMPORTANT REFERENCES ARE FOUND ON PAGE 211.

D.7. Basic Gross Motor Assessment (BGMA)

DESCRIPTION

The Basic Gross Motor Assessment[1,2] was developed to evaluate the gross motor performance of children by quantifying the quality of their movements. It attempts to discriminate between children with aberrations due to experiential lag versus those requiring medical referral due to a physical impairment. The BGMA was designed for clinical practice and for research.

Population	Time to Complete	Cost	Training
Children with minor motor dysfunction, aged 5 1/2 to 12 1/2 years.	Not indicated.	Not indicated.	No special training is required. Examiners must be familiar with the administration and scoring procedures.

INSTRUCTIONS

A description of the administration procedure for each of the items is provided. "Good" performance and possible deviations for each item are defined.

SCALING

Format

Task performance.

Subscales

The assessment consists of 9 gross motor tasks:

Standing balance on one leg, eyes open   Hopping on one foot
Standing balance on one leg, eyes closed   Skipping
Stride jump   Target throwing with bean bags
Tandem walking   Yo-yo
Ball handling

Scoring

Each item is scored on a 4-point ordinal scale (One point is subtracted for each deviation from the criteria for good performance):

3 - Good performance
2 - Fair (1 deviation)
1 - Poor (2 deviation)
0 - Unable to perform task or > 2 deviations

The assessment was standardized on 1,260 children aged 6-12 years, from 18 schools in the United States.

RELIABILITY

Internal consistency

The correlations between the split halves were calculated based upon 180 evaluations. The correlation for the total group was a moderate .71. Correlations for the individual ages were also moderate ranging from 0.59-0.79.[2]

Test-retest Reliability

Fourty-eight children were tested twice within a 2 day interval. The correlation between the 2 test scores was high (0.97).[2]

Interrater Reliability

Ten children were evaluated and rated by 5 observers. The correlation between the test results was high (0.97).[2]

VALIDITY

Content (domain or face)

A panel of professionals agreed on the face validity of the items included in the test.

Construct

A factor analysis[2] on the items of the BGMA revealed 7 factors:

Standing balance - eyes open
Elementary ball handling
Static balance - eyes closed
Leg strength and balance
Object control
Aiming
Dynamic balance

Concurrent

Physical education teachers rated students' abilities in physical education activities from high (5) to low (1). Correlations between the ratings and BGMA scores ranged up to 0.79.[2]

Predictive

Not reported.

Discriminative

The BGMA has the ability to discriminate between students and matched controls at 6 to 12 years of age. The 2 groups obtained significantly different scores (t = -3.47, p <.01).[2]

IMPORTANT REFERENCES ARE FOUND ON PAGE 212.

D.8. Bruininks – Oseretsky Test of Motor Proficiency (BOTMP)

DESCRIPTION

This Test is an adaptation of the Oseretsky Tests of Motor Proficiency and provides a comprehensive index divided into separate measures of gross motor and fine motor skills. The complete scale comprises 46 items but a short form, useful for screening, consists of only 14. The test has been used to identify and evaluate motor dysfunction in school age children. It was designed for both screening and for identifying physical problems in children, and has been used for planning and evaluation of motor training programs and as an aid in the decision making process for educational placement. It has also been used for screening of non-disabled children and the evaluation of children who are intellectually challenged or learning disabled. Examiners must be familiar with the administration and scoring procedures. It has been used by educators, psychologists, physical therapists and occupational therapists. Testing requires several basic items of equipment such as chairs, a mat, stop watch, and table.

Population	Time to Complete	Cost	Training
Children with minor motor dysfunction 4.5 to 14.5 years.	40 - 60 min.	The manual and test kit $250 U.S. (1984).	None required.

INSTRUCTIONS

The detailed manual describes all the materials needed, the directions for administering each item and the criteria for scoring.

SCALING

Format
Task performance.

Subscales

The test consists of 46 items divided into 8 subtests: 4 gross motor subtests, 1 upper limb test and 3 fine motor subtests. The subtests are combined into a fine motor and gross motor composite:

Gross Motor Composite	Fine Motor Composite
Running speed and agility (1 item)	Response speed (1 item)
Balance (8 items)	Visual-motor control (8 items)
Bilateral coordination (8 items)	Upper-limb speed and dexterity (8 items)
Strength (3 items)	Upper limb Coordination (9 items)

Scoring

Each item is scored on a variable scale ranging from 2 to 17 points.

Norms for various subgroups of children based on age, sex, race, community size and geographical region were generated using information collected on 765 children, selected from schools, day care centers, nursery schools and kindergartens in the U.S. and Canada.

Normalized standard scores for the Gross Motor Composite, Fine Motor Composite and the total Battery Composite have a mean of 50 and a standard deviation of 10. The subtest scores all have a mean of 15 and a standard deviation of 5.

Standardized scores (developed with all ages combined), percentile ranks, stanines and Z scores are provided. Age equivalent scores are available for each of the subtest scores.

RELIABILITY

Internal consistency

Ninety 8-year old and 90 12-year old children were assessed on the items comprising the subtests, the composite test and the short-form. The intercorrelations were highly variable[1] ranging from 0.00 to 0.93.

Test-retest Reliability

Sixty-three second grade and 63 sixth grade students were evaluated twice within 7 to 12 days. The results indicated a moderate to high correlation between the two test scores for the total Battery Composite (0.68-0.89). The results for the individual subtests were more variable (0.29-0.89).[1]

Interrater Reliability

Correlation coefficients of 0.9 to 0.98 were reported but no information is provided as the number of raters evaluating the number of subjects evaluated.[1]

VALIDITY

Content (domain or face)

Items were drawn form the Oseretsky Test of Motor Proficiency.

Construct

Thirty of the 60 Oseretsky items were selected for use in the BOTMP. An additional 70 items were added. An item analysis was performed using the test results from 75 children. Forty-six items were retained in the final version.[1]

The correlations of the test results with chronological age ranged from low to high, varying by subtest (0.57-0.86).

Test of internal consistency indicated that the correlations of the individual items with the subtest scores ranged from low to high (0.40-0.92), and for the total Battery Composite ranged from low to moderate (0.05-0.88).

Concurrent

Not reported.

Predictive

Not reported.

Discriminative

The test has the ability to discriminate between children of the same chronological age classified as mildly retarded, moderately to severely retarded, learning disabled, or normal.

IMPORTANT REFERENCES ARE FOUND ON PAGE 212.

D.9.　Gross Motor Function Measure (GMFM)

DESCRIPTION

The GMFM was developed to measure the presence or absence of change in the gross motor function of children with cerebral palsy in clinical practice and for research. Testing requires several basic items of equipment, such as toys, a mat, bench and a stop watch.[1-4] It may be used to describe a child's current level of function, to determine treatment goals, and to evaluate the effectiveness of therapies aimed at improving motor function.

Population	Time to Complete	Cost	Training
Cerebral palsy individuals, < 20 years of age (motor range up to 5 years).	45-60 minutes.	The test kit must be purchased $50 (1991).	Designated physical therapists. Further training to achieve criterion.

INSTRUCTIONS

The administration and scoring guidelines contain definitions for partial and complete achievement of each item.

SCALING

Format

Task performance.

Subscales

The test consists of 88 items divided into 5 dimensions. They are grouped by test position and arranged in developmental sequence:

Lying and Rolling: supine (9 items), prone (8 items)
Crawling and Kneeling: 4-point (14 items)
Sitting: (20 items)
Standing: (13 items)
Walking, Running, and Jumping: walking, kicking, jumping, climbing (24 items)

Scoring

Each item is scored on a 4-point ordinal scale:

0 - Cannot initiate task
1 - Initiates independently, completes < 10% of task
2 - Partially completes task, completes 10 to < 100% of task
3 - Completes task independently, 100%

Each child is first scored without and then with the orthosis or aid that is usually worn. A score for each of the 5 dimensions, as well as a total score, can be obtained. Each dimension provides a raw score, a percent score, and a total % score. A goal % score may be calculated, and refers to the % score for those areas that are treatment goals.

RELIABILITY

Internal consistency

Not reported.

Test-retest Reliability

Six therapists evaluated a total of 10 children representative of the ages and severities of cerebral palsy included in a study of 111 children. The therapists administered and scored the GMFM twice on the same child within a 2 week period. The ICC for the total score was high (-0.99). Individual dimensions ranged from 0.92 -0.99.[3]

Interrater Reliability

Six pairs of therapists evaluated 11 children representative of the ages and severities included in the larger study. The ICC for the total score was 0.99. Individual dimensions ranged from 0.87 - 0.99.[3]

VALIDITY

Content (domain or face)

Clinicians at 2 medical centers judged the test to have face validity. Item selection was based on a review of the literature and the judgement of clinicians at 3 medical centers. Items judged to be measurable, clinically important, and with the potential to show change in function were included.

Construct

Not reported.

Concurrent

One hundred and eleven children with cerebral palsy were evaluated twice over several months. The change scores were correlated with independent judgements of change in motor functions made by parents, therapists and blinded video observers. The GMFM correlated moderately with video-based evaluations (0.82) and poorly with therapists' judgement (0.65) and parents' judgement (0.54).

Predictive

Not reported.

Responsiveness

The GMFM is responsive to both negative and positive change. In a non-disabled population, those children younger than 3 years showed more change than those older than 3 years (t-test $p < .0001$). Those children with acute head injury improved significantly more than the non-disabled children, who improved more than those with cerebral palsy. (ANOVA $p < .05$).[3]

IMPORTANT REFERENCES ARE FOUND ON PAGE 212.

D.10. Gross Motor Performance Measure (GMPM)

DESCRIPTION

The GMPM is a measure of the <u>quality of movement</u> in children with cerebral palsy.[1-5] It was developed to be used in conjunction with the Gross Motor Function Measure which measures quantity. The GMPM can be used in clinical practice and research to profile the changes in movement quality.

Population	Time to Complete	Cost	Training
Children with cerebral palsy	Not reported.	Not reported.	Requires special training.

INSTRUCTIONS

Administration guidelines are available.

SCALING

Format

Task performance. Three of the 5 performance attributes are tested on each of 20 GMFM items.

Subscales

The assessment consists of 5 performance attributes.
1. Alignment - arrangement of body segments in relation to each other
2. Coordination - smooth use of movements
3. Dissociated movement - isolated movements
4. Stability - maintenance of body position
5. Weight shift - movement involving transfer of body's center of gravity

Scoring

A generic scoring scale rates each item on a 5-point scale, varying from severely abnormal to consistently normal. Performances are averaged to calculate a percent score for each attribute and an overall score. Minimum score 20%; maximum score 100%.

RELIABILITY

Internal consistency

Not reported.

Test-retest Reliability

Three pairs of physiotherapists tested 25 cerebral palsied and 5 normal children twice within two weeks. Reliability of attribute subscales ranged from ICC = 0.89 to 0.96; total ICC = 0.96. Confidence interval: 0.93 - 0.98.

Intrarater Reliability

Videotapes were scored on one occasion and again by the same therapists after 8 weeks. Reliability of subscales ranged from ICC = 0.90 to 0.97; total ICC = 0.93. Confidence interval: 0.92 to 0.98.

Interrater Reliability

Children were also assessed by two therapists (one handling, one observing). Reliability of subscales ranged from 0.84 to 0.94. Total ICC = 0.92. Confidence interval: 0.85 - 0.97.

VALIDITY

Content (domain or face)

A panel of 11 experts in developmental therapy and research judged the attributes, the test format and the scoring system. The revised version was sent to the panel for consensus, demonstrating that the GMPM has satisfactory clarity, completeness, and potential for evaluation of change.

Construct

Preliminary results of validation study show that the quality of movement in non-disabled children did not change significantly over a month's time frame while cerebral palsy children did change (p = 0.02) and head injured children changed a great deal (p = 0.006). Older children (7 to 12 years) changed more than younger children (0 to 2 years).[6]

Concurrent

Not reported.

Predictive

Not reported.

IMPORTANT REFERENCES ARE FOUND ON PAGE 213.

D.11. Movement Assessment of Infants (MAI)

DESCRIPTION

Developed as a screening tool to identify and evaluate motor dysfunction of high risk infants,[1-3] it can aid in establishing need for early intervention programs, and in monitoring the effects of physiotherapy. The evaluation techniques are helpful in teaching skillful observation of movement. It is not a measure of diagnosis or prediction. A normal profile has been developed for children 4 and 8 months of age. Training courses are available. The assessment is designed for use by professionals with a specialized knowledge of infant development.

Population	Time to Complete	Cost	Training
Children 0 to 12 mo (adjusted) at high risk for motor dysfunction.	Maximum 1.5 hours is necessary to test and score.	$9 manual. $3 for 50 scoresheets.	Formal training not required, but courses available.

INSTRUCTIONS

The manual provides excellent instructions to administer and score each item.

SCALING

Format

    Task performance.

Subscales

    The assessment consists of 65 items divided into four sections:
        Muscle tone (passive, active)
        Primitive reflexes
        Automatic reactions (righting, equilibrium, protective)
        Volitional movements

Scoring

    Each item in the muscle tone section is scored on a 6-point, bi-directional, ordinal scale, with " - " indicating normal tone, " > " high tone and " < " low tone. The remaining items are scored on a 4-point unidirectional scale, with 1 being the optimal or most mature response. The presence of asymmetry is also scored. The item responses are then matched against the high-risk profile for 4 or 8 month old infants, and each item is rated as either high-risk or normal. The number of high risk points for each of the sections and for the total assessment are used as the basis for evaluation and comparison.

RELIABILITY

Internal consistency

Not reported.

Test-retest Reliability

Twenty-seven full-term and 26 pre-term infants were evaluated twice within 7 days at 4 months of age by a total of 11 raters. The correlation between the total test scores was good (.76), but for subsections it varied (0.16-0.87) with volitional movement poorest.[4,5] Testing of 29 high and low risk infants at 4 months of age gave high Kappa scores (0.75-0.97).[4]

Interrater Reliability

Twenty-seven full-term and 26 pre-term infants were evaluated by 2 raters, at 4 months of age, with a moderate correlation for the total score (0.72). The subsection correlation ranged from poor to moderate (0.51-0.78), volitional movement being the least reliable.[4,5]

Fifty-three high and low risk infants were rated by 2 examiners at 4 months of age. Kappa statistics were fair to good (0.4-.07).[4]

VALIDITY

Content (domain or face): Not reported.

Construct: Not reported.

Concurrent

A total of 311 infants were evaluated at 4 months on the MAI and the Bayley Psychomotor Scale. Correlations between the test scores was moderate (-0.63).[6]

Predictive

Seventy-seven infants were evaluated on the MAI at 4 months and on the Peabody at 4.5 years. The correlations between the total scores on the two tests at different time points was poor (-0.12) and even lower for the divided subscales (-0.01 to 0.15).[3]

Several studies examined the predictive validity of the MAI. A large study of 152-4 month old infants, followed until age 3-8 years found the sensitivity of the MAI to detect a diagnosis of cerebral palsy was 63% and its specificity 74%.[7] Several of the individual items were found to be predictive of cerebral palsy.[8]

Two hundred and forty-six infants were tested on the MAI at 4 months. The MAI was a poor predictor of 1 year (0.36) and 2 year (0.37) Bayley motor scales.[6] The MAI was also found to be a poor predictor of $4\frac{1}{2}$ year Peabody Gross Motor Scores (-0.01-0.15).[3]

Discriminative

A group of 229 infants were evaluated at 4 months of age. The items discriminated between an outcome of cerebral palsy and non handicapped: 17 items $p. < 0.001$; 15 items $.01 < p < .05$.[7]

Responsiveness

Ten children with Down's Syndrome were evaluated on the MAI twice, 6 weeks apart. T-tests indicated a significant difference between the 2 testing times, indicating that the test was able to detect subtle changes in motor ability.

IMPORTANT REFERENCES ARE FOUND ON PAGE 213.

D.12. Pediatric Evaluation of Disability Inventory (PEDI)

DESCRIPTION

The PEDI was developed to provide a comprehensive clinical assessment of key functional capacities and performance in children between the ages of 6 months and 7 years. Functional performance is measured by the level of caregiver assistance needed to accomplish major functional activities.

Population	Time to Complete	Cost	Training
Children with disability with functional performance level under 7 years.	Dependent on format.	Manual $75 (US) Plus scoresheets $85 and software $185.	Specific training required.

INSTRUCTIONS

A detailed test manual "Pediatric Evaluation of Disability Inventory (PEDI): Development, Standardization and Administration Manual" may be bought from the PEDI Research Group, Department of Rehabilitation Medicine, New England Medical Center Hospital, 750 Washington Street, Boston, MA 02111-1901.

SCALING

Format

Parent report/structured interview, administration by professional judgement, or by a combination of methods.

Subscales

Measures both capacity and performance in 3 content domains: 1) self care (15 items), 2) mobility (14 items), 3) social function (12 items). There are 3 distinct measurement sections: 1) Functional skills checklist, 2) Caregiver assistance, and 3) Modification Scale.

Scoring

Items are scored on a 6-point scale with 0 = total assistance and 5 = independent. There is also a modification scale to indicate routinely needed modifications. Scores are recorded in a booklet which also contains a summary score sheet that can be used to construct a profile of the child's performance across the different domains and scales. A software program for data entry, scoring, and generation of profiles is also available.

RELIABILITY

Internal consistency

Coefficient alpha values range from 0.95 to 0.99. (Study sample n = 410 for functional skills and n = 401 for caregiver assistance.)[1]

Test-retest Reliability

Not yet completed.

Interrater Reliability

Between interviewer and family respondent ICC for subscales range from 0.30 (social function) to 0.95; for total function ICC = 0.95; for total caregiver assistance 0.96; and for total modifications 0.91.

VALIDITY

Content (domain or face)

Item selection was directed by the criterion of identifying meaningful functional units within complex functional activities.[1]

Construct

N/A.

Criterion

Concurrent validity was studied by comparing PEDI scores with the Battelle Developmental Inventory Screening Test and the Wee FIM. Values ranged from 0.66 to 0.93. Across similar content domains values ranged from 0.64 to 0.97.[1]

Responsiveness

The measure was found to be responsive in all domains for children with minor trauma, and in self care and mobility domains for children with severe disabilities.[1]

IMPORTANT REFERENCES ARE FOUND ON PAGE 214.

Now, are you ready? Here's your first chance to respond. The following pages are several "tear out" forms. For those of you who are "up" on your measures, use the blank template to review additional ones either for yourself and/or to return to us for future action. You can participate by helping us to update our information on the measures reviewed.

If you're not ready for that, then use the general feedback sheet to suggest either additional measures you'd like reviewed or to give your general recommendations of any kind.

MEASURE _____

DESCRIPTION

Population	Time to Complete	Cost	Training

INSTRUCTIONS

SCALING

Format

Subscales

Scoring

RELIABILITY

Internal consistency

Test-retest Reliability

Interrater/Intrarater Reliability

VALIDITY

Content (domain or face)

Construct

Criterion

Predictive

Responsiveness

HERE'S YOUR CHANCE TO RESPOND AND MAKE RECOMMENDATIONS

GENERAL FEEDBACK ON THE DOCUMENT

_____

_____

_____

_____

_____

_____

_____

_____

_____

_____

SUGGESTIONS FOR IMPROVEMENTS

_____

_____

_____

_____

_____

_____

_____

_____

_____

_____

Cont'd over

SUGGESTIONS CONT'D

_____

_____

_____

_____

_____

_____

_____

_____

FUTURE DIRECTION
(Where would you like us to go from here?)

_____

_____

_____

_____

_____

_____

_____

_____

Canadian Physiotherapy Association
890 Yonge Street, 9th Floor
Toronto, Ontario
M4W 3P4

Your Name, Address and Phone Number:
_____

_____

_____

_____

PART IV

Measuring Outcomes: Systems

If the **outcome measures** form the *"Heart of the Matter"* as proclaimed in the title of Part III, **Outcome Measurement Systems** form the *Circulatory System* for the living organism we are discussing. Until a systematic application of reliable, valid, standard measurements becomes routine in physical rehabilitation, we will not reach the potential to use these measures constructively to improve client care. Nor will we be able to use them to accurately differentiate between the treatments which are effective from those which are not.

We are far from being alone in this rapid evolution. Many professional groups are in various stages of maturation in similar efforts. For example, existing treatment methods in medicine and surgery are also under scrutiny. Driven by necessity in many cases, research clinicians and pharmaceutical companies have devised elaborate systems for testing new drugs for acute treatments. Some of the methodology used is quickly spreading from clinical epidemiology into clinical management of both acute and chronic medical conditions. Physical rehabilitation can also take advantage of these approaches to clinical decision making.

Scientifically established evidence should be driving health care decisions at all levels: clinical, administrative, regulatory, national policy, and research. But we know that this is often not so. Primary among the reasons are lack of sufficient measures and measurement systems that are psychometrically sound, and hence, adequate databases from which to derive reliable and valid guidelines for clinical practice.[1]

As Dr. Gonnella points out in the above quote, there are two major deficits with the information we get in the clinical setting – a lack of measures and measurement systems. The latter problem is the focus of this part of the book.

Despite the high level of interest in the measurement of outcomes, there is a general lack of knowledge of how to go about this complex process. From our survey we found that therapists want an understanding of the issues, knowledge of the properties of measures suitable for use in various specialties, and suggestions or guidelines for the implementation of a system for outcome measurement. Therefore, this part of our book will focus on the following:

Issues and Implementation Strategies

- current problems limiting use of outcome measurement

- purposes for measuring outcomes

- use of the International Classification for Impairment Disability and Handicap (ICIDH) framework

- outcome attributes

- selection of outcome measures

- adjustment for severity and other prognostic indicators

- application

CURRENT PROBLEMS

Problems associated with our current methods of evaluating health care have resulted in a growing interest in outcome measurement. The following seven concerns were articulated at the National Workshop on Patient Outcome Measures, Toronto, Canada, 1990.[2] Instead of lessening, the importance of each these concerns seems only to be increasing over time.

- Interventions are often not subjected to evaluation before they become common practice

- It is increasingly difficult to mount convincing arguments in favour of introducing new interventions and even maintaining many well established ones in the face of uncertainty and lack of consensus about their efficacy

- Our current quality assurance activities are not designed to give us a clear focus of what constitutes appropriate care

- Progress in outcome measurement has been impeded by assertions from health professionals that their clients are unique

- Outcomes are usually defined by the provider, not the clients — clients and caregivers. While the two may be complementary, they may not be the same

- Incentives in the health care system are working against us. Funding is volume driven, not quality driven

- Many health care professionals are threatened by outcome measurement

From the results of our survey, you saw that some of these problems continue to be barriers. We might add:

- Lack of understanding of the difference between evaluating the outcome of an individual client compared to evaluating outcome of a homogeneous group of clients

- A belief that a clinician's time is better spent in delivering client care of uncertain efficacy than in examining the relative efficacy of different treatments

- A belief that the time spent in identifying and administering outcome measures will not result in improved client care and therefore is not justified

PURPOSES FOR MEASURING OUTCOMES

The most important step in the process of developing a system for measuring outcomes is the careful consideration of the purpose or purposes for such a system. Too often when we consider these purposes we become overwhelmed – too many purposes, too much variability among clients, and too much diversity of clients' goals and abilities. Starting with a small and manageable list is often wise. Consider essential purposes only and document these purposes in detail. Examples of headings to consider when elucidating purposes include:

- clinical practice
- utilization review
- case management
- program evaluation
- quality management

During **clinical practice**, the client and therapist are interested in the effectiveness of individual treatment strategies in order to plan treatment and monitor the response of the individual. For example, outcomes in a client with low back pain undergoing a strengthening, flexibility and fitness program might be evaluated by the Oswestry Pain Disability Questionnaire, Modified Schober Test for spinal range of motion, hand-held dynamometer for strength testing of abdominals and back extensors, and Self-Paced Walk Test for aerobic capacity. Outcome measurement for this purpose tends to focus on specific components of function or impairments that are expected to change with treatment. The components measured are often discipline specific. The improvement of functional movement (walking) which is expected to improve as a result of the change in a component (range of motion or strength of a specific muscle group) should also be measured as it is usually of primary concern to the client. The improvement of functional movement may also be a multidisciplinary goal. The outcome measure used for this purpose should be highly sensitive to clinically important change. The information obtained is used concurrently and prospectively for that individual. In addition, aggregate standardized clinical assessment data of homogeneous client groups are useful in setting goals for similar individual clients in the future.

Utilization review addresses the pattern of use of services. Some efficiency measures are useful in this context to enable managers to determine resource allocation. Examples might be outcome measures which determine the relative effect of using different types of strength training equipment or those which compare the relative effect of a home program of treatment with regular attendance at a clinical facility for treatment. Efficiency measures such as hospital length of stay, use of medical or rehabilitation services, or compliance with a home program of exercises will provide information which will assist with utilization review.

Case management is usually accomplished in interprofessional rounds. The data collected by several professionals during the treatment period are used to evaluate that individual's progress and plan future treatment. These data can also contribute to program evaluation by providing data points between admission and discharge. We can frequently gain important information by measuring clients at several points during the treatment program to determine when the most change is made and when further treatment has minimal effect on physical function. These data can help us in decisions regarding treatment of individual clients but can also help us to tailor treatment programs to produce the best effect in clients in the most efficient way.

Program evaluation may focus on structure, process, or outcome to determine program effectiveness and efficiency. Increasingly, the measurement of the functional performance of clients has been included as an important outcome of rehabilitation programs. This usually involves global measurement of the outcomes of interest prior to the start of the program, at discharge and/or follow-up, and is often accomplished by a multiprofessional team. The information obtained is often used retrospectively to assist in future planning of the program but can also be used prospectively to determine expected change for future individual clients.

Quality management involves many procedures, protocols, and programs to improve the quality of care in a facility. Outcome measurement is one way of assessing the quality of care and the data generated can then be used to identify areas which need to be addressed to improve that care. Other aspects of quality assurance and/or quality management linked with outcome measurement may be **utilization review, risk management, case management, etc.**

USE OF THE ICIDH FRAMEWORK

The best framework for considering important outcomes is the International Classification for Impairment Disability and Handicap.[3] The terms used in this classification are defined in the accompanying box.

ESSENTIAL DEFINITIONS[3]

Impairment: is any loss or abnormality of psychological, physiological or anatomical structure or function.

Disability: is any restriction or lack of ability to perform an activity in a manner, or within the range, which is considered normal. Disability represents a departure from the norm in terms of performance of the individual, as opposed to that of an organ or mechanism.

Handicap: a disadvantage for a given individual, resulting from an impairment or a disability, that limits or prevents the fulfilment of a role that is normal for that individual (depending on age, sex, social and cultural factors).

Considering outcomes in these 3 domains can be very useful because, although the 3 parameters are related, each is unique. The relationship between the 3 is not linear – the magnitude of the handicap results not only from the interaction of the impairment and disability, but also from the individual's physical environment, social and economic setting and the resources available. The impairment outcomes are often the components of a particular function and each discipline has specific impairments it usually addresses in treatment (e.g. muscle strength or joint range of motion). Disability outcomes usually involve the whole person and are more often functional outcomes (e.g. walking velocity or walking distance). These are more often of primary concern to clients. Outcomes related to handicap frequently involve the individual's ability to interact with others and with the environment (e.g. to go to work regularly) and are also important to the client.

In addition to functional outcomes, "rehabilitation professionals may engage in activities aimed at goals outside the domain of most functional outcome measures (e.g. prevention of secondary complications, prevention of death, family education, arranging for attendants or housing). In summary, functional measures are useful and essential in a context that must include other measures and procedures pertinent to the specific aims and areas of practice."[4]

OUTCOME ATTRIBUTES

Before selecting outcome measures, it is important to consider the parameters or attributes that reflect the overall goals of treatment – from a client (or caregiver), professional, and public perspective.

For example, using the ICIDH framework, the most significant outcome attributes for the neurological area of practice (see box below) were identified at the National Outcome Measurement Workshops.[2] This list is not considered either exhaustive or definitive but provides an indication of attributes considered important to this area of practice.

OUTCOME ATTRIBUTES RELEVANT TO PHYSICAL ASPECTS OF NEUROLOGICAL DISEASE OR DISORDER[2]

Sensorimotor and Indirect Impairments

postural control	tone/spasticity	coordination
voluntary movements	range of motion	involuntary movements
(including gait)	strength	fitness
sensation		

Physical Disabilities

self care	mobility	arm & hand function
gross motor function	locomotion	burden on caregiver
	(including walking)	

Handicaps

return to role/productive participation
ability to cope/adjust to disability
empowered control over own life
satisfaction/quality of life
community integration/living arrangement

ADJUSTMENT FOR SEVERITY AND OTHER PROGNOSTIC INDICATORS

"Outcomes are highly affected by client severity at admission."[4] Levels of functional performance at admission may vary widely among individual clients. The strength gain expected in an individual who is debilitated by prolonged lack of normal activity will be very different from an individual who has a loss of strength due to a short period of interrupted training. As a result, comparison of simple gain scores (the score at discharge minus the score at admission) is a controversial issue. A change of 10 points at one point on a scale may have a different meaning clinically if the same amount of change occurs at another point on the scale. This becomes particularly problematical if the scale being used is ordinal as the change in 10 points at one position of the scale is not equal to the change of 10 points at another point on the scale.

Whether referred to as "risk adjustment" or "prognosis adjustment," consideration should be given to the factors that influence outcome variability. The identification of a set of significant prognostic variables can improve our precision with goal setting and our predictions of expected outcome. Examples of important prognostic variables include:

- severity of various impairments
- severity of various disabilities
- age
- co-morbidity/complications (e.g. incontinence)
- client attitudes, beliefs and expectations
- social factors/caregiver support/financial resources
- occupation
- duration and intensity of physical therapy and other health care services

The development of outcome prediction equations using the relevant prognostic variables can also improve our ability in goal setting and determining expected outcomes.

APPLICATION

Our survey conducted with Canadian physical therapists illustrates that clinicians are not looking for a single approach to outcome measurement. Rather, these managers and clinicians want information which can help in the selection of outcome measures and guidelines for setting up systems to apply these measures appropriately to their needs. The systems needed will vary depending upon purposes, settings and populations. Referring back to the purpose or purposes for which a system is needed, clinicians should consider whether a *single-case evaluation* or a *group application* is required. For single-case evaluation of outcomes, two methods are commonly used. The first is a simple change in score from one time of measurement to the next, using a standardized measure such as the disability inventory of the Chedoke-McMaster Stroke Assessment.[5] The second method is *Goal Attainment Scaling* (GAS) for which Palisano et al[6] provide an excellent example.

SINGLE-CASE EVALUATION

Use of Change/Gain Scores

Several alternatives are available:

1. *Choose the component and functional attributes which are expected to change with treatment in that individual.*

   This could be done by a therapist in collaboration with each individual treated, but most therapists will identify attributes of clinical importance for the groups of clients they usually work with and choose among them after discussion with the client about his/her goals. An alternative is for several therapists who work with a similar client population to combine their clinical judgement to decide the range of attributes they think are important to that client group and then choose from among these the ones most important to each individual client.

2. *Choose the best standardized measure available to measure each attribute.*

   A standardized measure is one which has been developed and tested for a specific purpose(s) in a specified population. Its psychometric properties have been tested to ensure the best method of scaling and scoring for the intended purpose. A manual or instructions have been published to enable the user to know exactly how the developers intend the test to be administered and the development and testing of the measure is reported in the literature. Some reliability and validity testing has been done. A standardized measure which is to be used as an outcome measure should have been tested for its responsiveness to clinically important change, an important feature for the validity of an outcome measure (See Part III.).

3. *Choose the appropriate times to administer the measure.*

   There must be a balance between too frequent administration which is frustrating to the client and is not time-efficient and too infrequent administration which may contribute to ineffective treatments being prolonged.

4. *Analyze results and provide feedback to the client.*

   The change/gain score should be compared to that expected during the treatment interval and conclusions regarding continuation or change of treatment discussed with the client. The expected change should, if possible, be based on a database for a similar population or on aggregate clinical data in conjunction with clinical judgement by the therapist related to the needs of that individual. Ideally a prediction equation for similar clients has been developed and can be used to determine expected outcome with adjustment for prognostic variables.

Use of Goal Attainment Scaling

Again, several alternatives are available:

1. *Choose component and functional attributes which are expected to change with treatment in that individual.*

    There is often one function or disability that is of primary importance to the client and becomes the goal of treatment. Next, specific components which are limiting that function are identified. For example, if ambulation outdoors is important to the client, the components might be level of pain during walking, balance, quadriceps strength, and hip range of motion.

2. *Identify what behaviours or outcomes will indicate expected change as a result of the treatment.*

    Indicators of behaviours need to be described in a specific measurable way. The client's present ability would be measured in the function and each of its components. Then the expected level of performance of each function and component after a specified time of treatment would be estimated. Ideally this estimate will be based on data from similar clients. For example, expected ambulation outdoors after 4 weeks of treatment might be ambulation at 80 meters/minute for a distance of 500 meters. Similarly the expected level of change for each of the components would be identified and they may be priorized on the basis of their importance in achieving the functional goal. If there are more than one functional goal, these may also be priorized by difficulty and/or importance to the client.

3. *Identify the most favourable and least favourable outcome for each goal and determine the intermediate levels of scaling.*

    Goal attainment scaling is traditionally measured on a 5-point scale with the expected outcome at the mid-point and 2 levels of greater than expected outcome and 2 levels below expected outcome. These must be written so that each level is measurable, with no gaps or overlaps in performance between levels.

4. *Determine how frequently goal attainment will be measured.*

    Similar to using change scores for outcome measurement, goal attainment measurement should be often enough to record clinically significant change when it occurs and not so frequent as to be discouraging for the client.

Goal attainment can be combined with program evaluation whereby one or two goals are chosen for all program participants in addition to individual goals which may be different. Program goals may only be measured at the start and end of the program and possibly for follow-up purposes.

Goal attainment scaling has the advantage of a measurement method which takes into account individual client differences while still allowing some comparison among homogeneous clients. The setting of the goals and describing of the levels takes skill to provide a reliable and valid measure.

Both goal attainment scaling and change scores can be used successfully in evaluating outcomes in individual clients. Each has advantages and limitations. For more information, see Palisano,[6] Malec et al,[7] and Ottenbacher and Cusick.[8]

GROUP EVALUATION

For program evaluation or quality improvement, a group application system is usually needed. Two types of systems suitable for this purpose are a database such as that designed by Haley et al,[9] and a "multi-facility" data system such as the Uniform Data System for medical Rehabilitation (UDS).[10] Systems such as the UDS allow a rehabilitation program to see how it compares with similar programs on "functional outcomes, functional gain, length of stay, and other basic factors."[4]

Our development of a database for the purpose of evaluation of groups first involves defining the objectives of the evaluation, only one of which may be documenting clinical outcomes. The client population must next be described including subgroups within the population, if applicable. The expected outcomes of the program for the total population or subgroup are next described. This can be done in terms of a level of performance or a percentage of change expected in each attribute. The expected outcome is completed for all program participants in addition to individual outcomes specific to each client.[9]

Specific standardized measures must next be chosen for each of the identified program objectives. (See Part III for criteria by which a range of possible measures can be evaluated.) The database must be carefully designed to be useful to therapists for individual and group decision-making and allow for easy collection, storage and retrieval of information.[9]

Once the implementation of a system is put into place careful consideration must be given to the summarization of the data output. Again, we must think back to the original purpose or purposes, to keep the process simple and to produce reports that provide data of use in our decision making.

The data that come from an outcome measurement system must always be put into context. These data can only provide information which <u>aids</u> in decision making. Decisions on the meaning of the data and the implications on future action require judgement if the ultimate purpose of determining the benefits of the services we provide is to be met.

PART V

THE X-ROADS

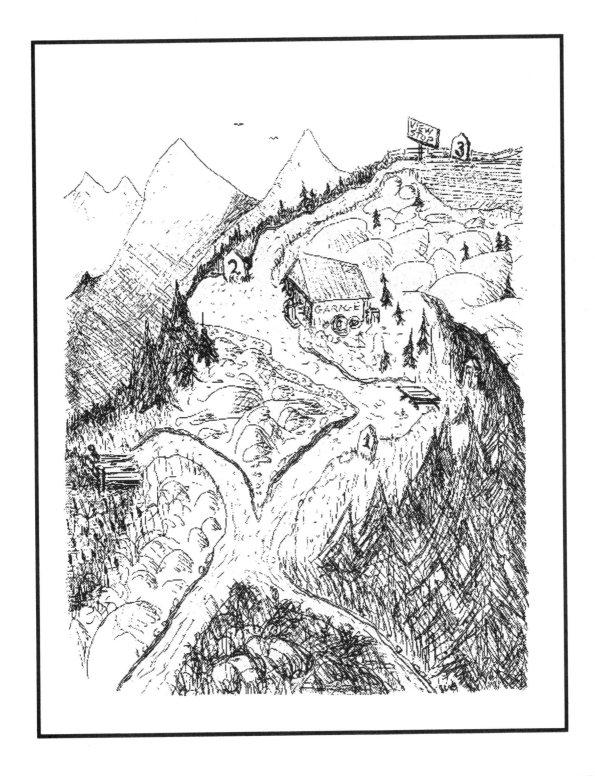

The challenge is to know where to go from here with the implementation of physical rehabilitation outcome measures. Based on the survey reported in Part II, our challenge was to decrease some of the barriers to the use of outcome measures. We also wished to facilitate their use by increasing knowledge of existing instruments and knowledge of instrument development.

We hope that Parts III and IV have, to some degree, addressed your knowledge of existing instruments and their development. In addition, we hope you have increased your understanding of how outcome measures can be implemented with individual clients as well as with groups of clients. What action can we now take on implementing some of these ideas in our own practice?

"Milestone 1"

"Milestone 1" marks an open-minded attitude to changes that are needed to implement outcome measures in a way that enhances:

a) the information and the treatment we can offer individual clients

b) the programs we can offer groups of clients with similar impairments, disabilities and handicaps.

This attitude involves acceptance of the necessity for standardized outcome measures in gathering information about clients in a systematic way.

"Milestone 2"

"Milestone 2" marks a change in our individual behaviour from whatever point we are, to the next step in the process of implementing outcome measures and using the information gained in the process for clinical decision making. For some of us, this will involve both identifying a standardized measure appropriate to assessing outcome in our clients and starting to collect these data systematically. For others, it will involve identifying other facilities who see a similar clientele to our own in order to pool data from a common standardized outcome measure. In this way information can be obtained from a larger group of clients more quickly. Some of us may well have collected the data with a suitable instrument already but need to start using these data. This would enable us to inform our clients about their progress and quantify more accurately the type or timing of changes that are occurring. We may also need to reconsider how we report these data to our colleagues and administrators for both clinical and administrative decisions. No doubt, with increased use of outcome measurement, we will become very aware of aspects of client's physical function which appear to be affected by treatment, but for which we have no standardized measure. In these instances, we need to challenge academic and clinical research colleagues to join us in adapting existing measures or developing and testing new measures to address these deficits. Each of us can choose where we wish to start changing our way of using outcome measurement; the important challenge is that we progress to the next step from whatever point we are at right now.

"Milestone 3"

"Milestone 3" involves the challenge for all of us who work in the area of physical rehabilitation:

A GENERAL ACCEPTANCE AND USE IN PHYSICAL REHABILITATION OF REGULAR MEASUREMENT OF THERAPEUTIC OUTCOMES USING PROVEN STANDARDIZED OUTCOME MEASURES.

Basic standards for users of outcome measures include:

- selecting the appropriate measure for a given population based on scientific evidence
- administering the measure according to the developers' procedure
- interpreting the results consistent with evidence of reliability and validity, and comparison to empirically derived norms of comparison group.

Clinicians, managers, educators, students, researchers, and consultants are all involved in meeting this challenge. In order to reduce the barriers and facilitate the implementation of outcome measurement, those playing each of these roles in physical rehabilitation will need to change attitudes and behaviour.

For clinicians, who consider themselves primarily users of outcome measures, the challenge will be to:

- increase the use of standardized outcome measures
- follow standards recommended for users in Appendix A and page 32 in Part III
- share data and results with others working with similar populations
- use the data gathered to improve the service provided to clients
- work with others to identify the need for improved measures

For directors and managers, the challenge will be to:

- value outcome measurement as an integral part of providing cost-effective care
- ensure that users of outcome measures in their departments apply appropriate standards
- encourage within and between-facility use of data including development of computer systems

- convince administrators and funding agencies that the information provided by the use of outcome measures is critical for decisions about competing resource allocation
- provide that information in a readily usable form

For educators, the challenge is to:

- facilitate the learning of the importance and use of outcome measurement as a necessary part of providing high quality client care by those entering the rehabilitation professions
- provide critical reviews of existing outcome measures in all areas of rehabilitation
- contribute toward the identification of areas where further development of measures are needed

For students, the challenge is to:

- understand the use of outcome measures in all aspects of rehabilitation practice
- become agents of change as they start work in facilities where outcome measurement has not become the accepted norm
- stay current with the growing literature on standardized outcome measurement

For researchers, the challenge is to:

- contribute to the identification of needed areas for new outcome measures
- lead in the adaptation and development of innovative, clinically useful outcome measures in all areas of rehabilitation

For administrators in government agencies, community facilities, rehabilitation centres, acute care and convalescent hospitals, home care and long term care centres, the challenge is to play their part in the change in attitudes and practice. No doubt when this is widely achieved there will be other uses and aspects to develop which we cannot envision at present. For the moment, let's each work toward this goal in whatever way we can. In this way we can all contribute to a broad acceptance of outcome measurement to improve the care we provide our clients.

NOT AN END BUT A BEGINNING

The challenge is clear and the opportunity is great. Together, we can make real progress reaching "Milestone 3" and beyond.

Your active participation is needed now. You can start (a) by using the tear-out template between page 158 and page 159 both for your own use and/or as a "mailer" to us, and (b) by completing the general feedback sheet.

APPENDIX A

Standards for Test Users

1. Persons should not become test users unless they are prepared to adhere to the Standards and understand the requirements for test purveyors.

2. Test users must have a basic understanding of local, state and federal laws governing the use of tests in their practice settings.

3. Test users must have a basic knowledge of the theory and principles of tests and measurements.

4. Test users must have background knowledge in basic, applied and clinical sciences related to the selection, administration, and interpretation of each test they use.

5. Test users must understand the theoretical bases (construct and content validity) for the tests they use, and they must have knowledge about the attribute (characteristics) being measured.

6. Test users must be familiar with the development of tests they use and the test settings in which those test have been developed and used.

7. Test users must understand how a test they are using relates to a similar test or previous versions of the same test.

8. Test users must be able to justify the selection of tests they use. Test users must also be prepared to supply logical arguments to justify the rejection of tests they choose not to use.

9. Test users must be able to identify their sources of information regarding tests they use. Test users must be able to specify where they obtained information (e.g. rationale and directions) for selecting and conducting a test.

10. Test users must understand all operational definitions related to tests they use.

11. Test users must be able to describe the population for whom the test was designed. Test users must be able to relate this description to the persons they are testing.

12. Test users must be able to determine before they use a test whether they have the ability to administer that test. This determination should be based on and understanding of the test user's own skills and knowledge (competency) as compared with the competencies described by the test purveyor.

13. Test users must follow instructions provided by purveyors for all tests they administer.

14. Test users must know what information and instructions are to be given to the person being tested. Test users should be able to answer questions about the test and related subjects.

15. Test users must know the physical settings in which the test should be given and the possible effects of conducting the test in other settings.

16. Test users must be able to identify any conditions or behaviors in the person being tested that may compromise the reliability or validity of their measurements (e.g. if a modified position must be used in manual muscle testing because of a deformity). Test users who observe such conditions or behaviors should note these observations in their reports of any resultant measurements. Test users who believe that the effect on their measurement could be significant should include a discussion on the implications of these observations in their reports.

17. Test users must have a basic understanding of the instruments they use as part of a test.

18. Test users must know how to use any instruments required to obtain the desired measurements. This standard includes, where appropriate, the test user knowing how to choose machine settings and other user-selected options. Test users must be able to discuss the effects of all options on their measurements and the consequences of selecting the incorrect options.

19. Test users must be able to describe how instruments they use for a test are calibrated, including the means of testing calibration. Test users must know the course of action to be taken when calibration is needed.

20. Test users, for all the tests they use, should be able to describe variations in the test procedures that are available. Test users must be able to describe variations that are known to impair the quality of the measurements and those variations that are known to lead to measurements of questionable validity.

21. Test users who deviate from accepted directions for obtaining a measurement should not use published data for documentation relative to reliability and validity to justify their use of the measurement.

22. Test users have a responsibility to suggest further testing when they have serious concerns about the quality of the measurement they obtain or when they believe that other test or other personnel can be used to obtain better measurements.

23. Test users who are required to derive or transform measurements must have sufficient training and knowledge to derive or transform those measurements. Test users must have the background information and skills needed to derive measurements or make categorizations necessary for interpretation of their measurements (e.g. how to normalize or standardize a score or how to classify a measurement).

24. Test users must be aware of any normative data for the measurements they are obtaining. Test users should be able to evaluate critically normative data and use the data for clinical decision making.

25. Test users must make every effort to control the environment (test setting) in which they test, in order to maintain consistent conditions between tests. These efforts are needed to ensure that the validity and reliability of a measurement are not compromised.

26. Test users must make every effort when personal information is being obtained to control the environment (test setting) in which they administer tests in order to preserve the privacy of the person taking the test.

27. Test users must be able to discuss common errors in the interpretation of the measurements they use.

28. Test users must make every effort to minimize the effect of reactivity associated with the tests they use.

29. Test users should report to the purveyor of the test any problems regarding a test or any associated instruments.

30. Test users should communicate with other test users and purveyors regarding their experience with tests.

31. Test users must avoid giving persons prior knowledge about the nature of a test when such knowledge is known to compromise the validity of the measurements.

32. Test users are responsible for maintaining confidentiality of test results. Confidentiality of results should be in accordance with standard practices in the institution or community in which the test user obtains the measurements. Results should not be shared with any persons (or organizations) who are known to be unwilling to respect the right of confidentiality for the person who was tested.

33. Test users should not share results with persons (or organizations) who are likely to misuse that information.

34. Test users must respect the rights of persons whom they test.

35. Test users must maintain records in such manner that information about tests and measurements is accurate and is not likely to be distorted or lost. Abbreviations used in communications should be limited to those that appear in established references.

36. Test users have a responsibility to report inappropriate test use to proper authorities.

37. Test users should select tests based on what is best for the person being tested. Test selection based on considerations of personal benefit to the test user, test purveyor, or the referring practitioner is inappropriate.

38. Test users, in clinical practice, should avoid the use of tests that were designed solely for research purposes. Such tests, when they are used in the clinical setting, should be identified in all reports as research tests that have not necessarily been shown to be reliable or valid in clinical use.

39. Test users should not assign persons to conduct tests unless they know that such persons are qualified to conduct the tests.

40. Test users should not make promotional claims for their testing procedures that are not supported by research literature.

41. Test users should assist in the development and refinement of testing procedures by sharing their knowledge of tests and assisting in the collection of data where appropriate.

42. Test users have a responsibility to periodically review the test procedures they and their colleagues use in their institutions (practice settings) to ensure the appropriate use of measurement is being made and that the rights of persons tested are being observed.

43. Test users who use tests that do not meet the Standards should be aware that these tests do not meet the Standards. Test users, therefore, should interpret results of these tests with caution and share these reservations with all persons who receive test results.

44. Test users must follow the basic rules and principles of measurement when they interpret results of tests they use.

45. Test users reporting the results of tests must supply adequate information so that these results can be understood.

REFERENCES

REFERENCES FOR ACKNOWLEDGEMENTS

1. Health and Welfare Canada. *Toward Assessment of Quality of Care in Physiotherapy.* Ottawa: Government of Canada 1980.

2. Health and Welfare Canada. *Toward Assessment of Quality of Care in Physiotherapy Volume II. Instruments to Measure Health Status of Patients Receiving Physiotherapy.* Ottawa: Government of Canada 1981.

REFERENCES FOR PART I

1. World Health Organization (WHO). *International Classification of Impairments, Disabilities and Handicaps. A manual of classification relating to the consequences of disease.* Geneva: World Health Organization, 1980.

2. Issues & Recommendations from the Proceedings of the National Workshop on Patient Care Outcome Measures. Don Mills, Ontario: Hospital Medical Records Institute 1991.

3. Canadian Council on Health Facilities Accreditation. *Quality Asurance: the Future.* Ottawa 1990.

4. Health and Welfare Canada. *Toward Assessment of Quality of Care in Physiotherapy Volume II: Instruments to Measure Health Status of Patients Receiving Physiotherapy.* Ottawa: Government of Canada 1981.

5. Johnston MV, Keith RA, Hinderer SR. Measurement standards for interdisciplinary medical rehabilitation. *Arch Phys Med Rehabil* 1992: 73: s3-s23.

6. Hayley SM, Baryza MJ, Lewin MJ, Cioffi MI. Sensorimotor dysfunction in children with brain injury: development of a data base for evaluation research. *Physical and Occupational Therapy in Pediatrics* 1991: 11(3): 1-26.

7. Keith RA, Granger CV, Hamilton BB, Sherwin FS. Functional Independence Measure. *Advances in Clinical Rehabilitation* 1987: 1: 6-18.

8. Mahoney FI, Barthel DW. Functional evaluation: the Barthel Index. *Maryland State Medical Journal* 1965: 14: 61-65.

9. McDowell I, Newell C. *Measuring Health: A Guide to Rating Scales and Questionnaires.* New York: Oxford Press 1987.

REFERENCES FOR PART III

INTRODUCTION TO PART III

1. Johnston MV, Keith RA, Hinderer SR. Measurement standards for interdisciplinary medical rehabilitation. *Arch Phys Med Rehabil* 1992: 73: s3-s23.

2. American Physical Therapy Association's Task Force on Standards for Measurement in Physical Therapy . Standards for tests and measurements in physical therapy practice. *Phys Ther* 1991: 71(8): 589-622.

3. Kirshner B, Guyatt G. A methodological framework for assessing health indices. *J Chronic Dis* 1985: 38(1): 27-36.

4. Guyatt GH, Feeny DH, Patrick DL. Measuring health-related quality of life. *Ann Intern Med* 1993: 118: 622-629

5. McDowell I, Newell C. *Measuring Health: A Guide to Rating Scales and Questionnaires*. New York: Oxford Press 1987.

6. Streiner DL, Norman GR. *Health Measurement Scales: a Practical Guide to their Development and Use*. New York: Oxford University Press 1989.

7. Law M. Measurement in occupational therapy: scientific criteria for evaluation. *Can J Occup Ther* 1987: 54(3): 133-138.

8. Weiner EA, Stewart BJ. *Assessing Individuals*. Boston: Little Brown 1984.

9. Burdick RK, Graybill FA. *Confidence Intervals on Variance Components*. New York: Marcel Dekker Inc. 1992: 126-131.

10. Bartko JJ, Carpenter WT. On the methods and theory of reliability. *The Journal of Nervous and Mental Disease* 1976: 163(5): 307-317.

11. Jaeschke R, Singer J, Guyatt GH. Measurement of health status. ascertaining the minimal clinically important difference. *Controlled Clin Trials* 1989: 10: 407-415.

REFERENCES FOR A. ADULT MOTOR AND FUNCTIONAL ACTIVITY MEASURES

A.1.   Timed "Up and Go"

1.   Podsiadlo D, Richardson S. The timed "up and go": A test of basic functional mobility for frail elderly persons. *Journal of the American Geriatrics Society* 1991: 39: 142-148.

2.   Mathias S, Nayak USL, Isaacs B. Balance in elderly patients: the "get-up and go" test. *Arch Phys Med Rehabil* 1986: 67: 387-389.

A.2.   Modified Sphygomomanometer for measuring muscle strength ("Modified Sphyg")

1.   Helewa A, Goldsmith C, Smythe H. The modified sphygmomanometer: A instrument to measure muscle strength: A validation study. *J Chronic Dis* 1981: 34: 353-361.

2.   Helewa A, Goldsmith C, Smythe H, Gibson E . An evaluation of four different measures of abdominal strength: patient, order and instrument variation. *Journal of Rheumatology* 1990: 17-7: 965-969.

3.   Giles C. The modified sphygmomanometer: an instrument to objectively assess muscle strength. *Physiother Can* 1984: 36: 36-41.

A.3.   Activity Index

1.   Stott DH, Moyes FA, Henderson SE. *Test of Motor Impairment*. Guelph, Ontario: Brook Educational Publishing Limited 1972.

A.4.   Motor Assessment Scale (MAS)

1.   Carr JH, Shepherd RB, Nordholm L, Lynne D. Investigation of a new motor assessment scale for stroke patients. *Phys Ther* 1985: 65: 175-178.

2.   Poole JL, Whitney SL. Motor assessment scale for stroke patients: concurrent validity and interrater reliability. *Arch Phys Med Rehabil* 1988: 69: 195-197.

3.   Lowen SC, Anderson BA. Reliability of the modified motor assessment scale and the Barthel Index. *Phys Ther* 1988: 68: 1077-1081.

4.   Lowen SC, Anderson BA. Predictors of stroke outcome using objective measurement scales. *Stroke* 1990: 21: 78-81.

Other Reading

Katrak PH, Cole AMD, Poulis CJ, McCauley JCK. Objective assessment of spasticity, strength, and function with early exhibition of dantrolene sodium after cerebovascular accident: a randomized double blind study. *Arch Phys Med Rehabil* 1992: 73: 4-9.

Shutter LA, Edwards DI, Wolf SL. Opinions and comments: new motor assessment scale examined. *Phys Ther* 1985: 65 (7):1091-1093.

A.5.   Chedoke-McMaster Stroke Assessment (Chedoke)

1.   Gowland C, Stratford P, Ward M, Moreland J, Torresin W, Van Hullenaar S, et al. Measuring physical impairment and disability with the Chedoke-McMaster Stroke Assessment. *Stroke* 1993: 24 (1): 58-63.

2.   Gowland C, Torresin W, Ward M, Stratford P. *Stroke rehabilitation: Validation of a physical impairment and disability measure*. Hamilton: McMaster Press 1993.

A.6.   Action Research Arm Test

1.   Carroll D. A quantitative test of upper extremity function. *Journal of Chronic Disability* 1965: 18: 479-491.

2.   Lyle RC. A performance test for assessment of upper limb function in physical rehabilitation treatment and research. *Inter J Rehabil Res* 1981: 4: 483-492.

3.   de Weerdt WJG, Harrison MA. Measuring recovery of arm-hand function in stroke patients: a comparison of the Brunnstrom-Fugl-Meyer test and the action research arm test. *Physiother Can* 1985: 37 (2): 65-70.

A.7.   Berg Balance Scale

1.   Berg KO, Wood-Dauphinee SL, Williams JI, Gayton D. Measuring balance in the elderly: preliminary development of an instrument. *Physiother Can* 1989: 41 (6): 304-311.

2.   Berg KO, Williams JI, Wood-Dauphine SL, Maki BE. Measuring balance in the elderly: validation of an instrument. *Canadian Journal of Public Health* 1992: 83: suppl. 7-11.

3.   Berg KO, Maki BE, Williams JI, Holliday PJ, Wood-Dauphine SL. Clinical and laboratory measures of postural balance in an elderly population. *Arch Phys Med Rehabil* 1992: 73: 1073-1080.

A.8. The Barthel Index

1. Mahoney FI, Barthel DW. Functional evaluation: The Barthel Index. *Maryland State Medical Journal* 1965: 14: 61-65.

2. Granger CV, Albrecht GL, Hamilton BB. Outcome of comprehensive medical rehabilitation: measurement by PULSES profile and the Bartel Index. *Arch Phys Med Rehabil* 1979: 60: 145-154.

3. Granger CV, Hamilton BB. Measurement of stroke rehabilitation outcome in the 1980s. *Stroke* 1990: 21: 46-47.

4. Granger CV, Greer DS, Liset E, Coulombe J, O'Brien E. Measurement of outcomes of care for stroke patients. *Stroke* 1975: 6: 34-41.

5. Granger CV, Hamilton BB, Gresham GE, Kramer AA. The stroke rehabilitation outcome study: part II. Relative merits of the total Barthel index score and a four-item subscore in predicting patient outcomes. *Arch Phys Med Rehabil* 1989: 70: 100-103.

6. Granger CV, Hamilton BB, Gresham GE. The stroke rehabilitation outcome study: Part 1. General description. *Arch Phys Med Rehabil* 1988: 69: 506-509.

7. Carter LT, Oliveira DO, Suptone J, Lynch SV. The relationship of cognitive skills performance to activities of daily living in stroke patients. *AJOT* 1988: 42: 449-445.

8. Chester CS, McLaren CE. Somatosensory evoked response and recovery from stroke. *Arch Phys Med Rehabil* 1989: 70: 520-525.

9. Chino N. Efficacy of Barthel Index in evaluating activites of daily living in Japan, the United States and United Kingdom. *Stroke* 1990: 21: 64-67.

10. Dejong G, Branch LG. Predicting the stroke patient's ability to live independently. *Stroke* 1982: 13: 648-655.

11. Gibson L, MacLennan WJ, Gray C, Pentland B. Evaluation of a comprehensive assessment battery for stroke patients. *Inter J Rehabil Res* 1991: 14: 93-100.

12. McGinnis GE, Seward ML, Dejong G, Osberg JS. Program evaluation of physical medicine and rehabilitation departments using self-report Barthel. *Arch Phys Med Rehabil* 1986: 67: 123-125.

13. Skyhoj OT. Arm and leg paresis as outcome predictors in stroke rehabilitation. *Stroke* 1990: 21: 247-251.

14. Ostrow P, Parents R, Ottenbacher KJ, Bonder B. Functional outcome and rehabilitation: An acute care field study. *J Rehabil Res Dev* 1989: 26: 17-26.

15. Roth E, Davidoff G, Haughton J, Ardner M. Functional assessment in spinal cord injury: a comparison of the Modified Barthel Index and the adapted Functional Independence Measure. *Clinical Rehabilitation* 1990: 4: 277-285.

16. Shah S, Vanclay F, Cooper B. Improving the sensitivity of the Barthel index for stroke rehabilitation. *J Clin Epidemiol* 1989: 42 (8): 703-709.

17. Wade DT, Skilbeck CE, Hewer RL. Predicting Barthel ADL score at 6 months after an acute stroke. *Arch Phys Med Rehabil* 1983: 64: 24-28.

18. Wylie CM. Measuring end results of rehabilitation of patients with stroke. *Public Health Rep* 1967: 82: 893-898.

19. Wylie CM, White BK. A measure of disability. *Arch Phys Med Rehabil* 1964: 8: 834-839.

20. Roy CW, Togneri J, Hay E, Pentland B. An inter-rater reliability study of the Barthel Index. *Inter J Rehabil Res* 1988: 11: 67-70.

21. Shinar D, Gross CR, Mohr JP, Caplan LR, Price TR, Wolf PA. Inter-observer variability in the assessment of neurologic history and examination in the stroke data bank. *Arch Neurol* 1985: 42: 557-565.

A.9. Functional Independence Measure (FIM)

1. Granger CV, Cotter A, Hamilton BB, Fiedler R, Hens MM. Functional assessment scales: a study of persons with multiple sclerosis. *Arch Phys Med Rehabil* 1990: 71: 870-875.

2. Granger CV, Hamilton BB, Keith RA, Zielezny M, Sherwins FS. Advance in functional assessment for medical rehabilitation. *Topics in Geriatric Rehabilitation* 1986: 1 (3): 59-74.

3. Keith RA, Granger CV, Hamilton BB, Sherwins FS. The Functional Independence Measure. *Advances in Clinical Rehabilitation* 1987: 1: 6-18.

4.   Roth E, Davidoff G, Haughton J, Ardner M. Functional assessment in spinal cord injury: a comparison of the Modified Barthel Index and the adapted Functional Independence Measure. *Clinical Rehabilitation* 1990: 4: 277-285.

5.   Whiteneck GG. A functional independence measure trial in SCI Model Systems. *American Spinal Injury Association Proceedings* 1982: 48.

A.10. The Fugl-Meyer Assessment of Sensorimotor Recovery After Stroke

1.   Fugl-Meyer AR. Post-stroke hemiplegia assessment of physical properties. *Scand J Rehabil Med* 1980: 7: 85-93.

2.   Duncan PW, Propst M, Nelson SG. Reliability of the Fugl-Meyer assessment of sensorimotor recovery following cerebrovascular accident. *Phys Ther* 1983: 63: 1606-1610.

3.   DiFabio RP, Badke MB. Relationship of sensory organization to balance function in patients with hemiplegia. *Phys Ther* 1990: 70 (9): 542-548.

4.   Berglund K, Fugl-Meyer AR. Upper extremity function in hemiplegia: a cross validation study of two assessment methods. *Scand J Rehabil Med* 1986: 18: 155-157.

5.   Clarke B, Gowland C, Brandstater M, deBruin H. A re-evaluation of the Brunnstrom assessment of motor recovery of the lower limb. *Physiother Can* 1983: 35 (4): 207-211.

Other Reading

de Weerdt WJG, Harrison MA. Measuring recovery of arm-hand function in stroke patients: a comparison of the Brunnstrom-Fugl-Meyer test and the action research arm test. *Physiother Can* 1985: 37 (2): 65-70.

Fugl-Meyer AR, Jaasko L, Leyman I, Olsson S, Steglind S. The post-stroke hemiplegic patient. I: a method for evaluation of physical performance. *Scand J Rehabil Med* 1975: 7: 13-31.

Kursoffsky A, Wadell I, Nilsson BY. The relationship between semsory impairment and motor recovery in patients with hemiplegia. *Scand J Rehabil Med* 1982: 14: 27-32.

Lindmark B, Hamrin E. Evaluation of functional capacity after stroke as a basis for active intervention: validation of a modified chart for motor capacity assessment. *Scand J Rehabil Med* 1988: 20: 111-115.

Twitchell TE. The restoration of motor function following hemiplegia in man. *Brain* 1951: 74: 443-480.

A.11. Katz Index of Activities of Daily Living

1.   Staff of the Benjamin Rose Hospital. Multidisciplinary studies of illness in aged persons: II. A new classification of functional status in activities of daily living. *J Chronic Dis* 1959: 9 (1): 55-62.

2.   Brorsson B, Asberg KH. Katz Index of Independence in ADL: reliability and validity in short-term care. *Scand J Rehabil Med* 1984: 16: 125-132.

3.   Asberg KH, Nydevik I. Early prognosis of stroke outcome by means of Katz Index of activities of daily living. *Scand J Rehabil Med* 1991: 23: 187-191.

4.   Gresham GE, Phillips TF, Wolf PA, McNamara PM, Kannel WB, Dawber TR. Epidemiologic profile of long-term stroke disability: The Framingham Study. *Arch Phys Med Rehabil* 1979: 60: 487-491.

Other Reading

Donaldson SW, Wagner CC, Gresham GE. A unified ADL evaluation form. *Arch Phys Med Rehabil* 1973: 54: 175-179.

Katz S, Ford AB, Moskowitz RW, Jackson BA, Jaffe MW. Studies of illness in the ages: The index of ADL: A standard measure of biological and psychosocial function. *Journal of the American Medical Association* 1963: 185: 914-919.

Staff of the Benjamin Rose Hospital. Multidisciplinary studies of illness of aged persons: III. Prognostic indices in fracture of hip. *J Chronic Dis* 1960: 11: 445-455.

Steinberg FU. The Stroke Registry: A prospective method of studying stroke. *Arch Phys Med Rehabil* 1973: 54: 31-35.

A.12. Kenny Self-Care Evaluation

1.   Grodeon EE, Drenth V, Jarvis L, Johnson J, Wright V. Neurophysiologic syndromes in stroke as predictors of outcomes. *Arch Phys Med Rehabil* 1978: 59: 399-409.

2.	Kerner JF, Alexander J. Activities of daily living: reliability and validity of gross vs specific ratings. *Arch Phys Med Rehabil* 1981: 62: 161-166.

3.	Donaldson SW, Wagner CC, Gresham GE. A unified ADL evaluation form. *Arch Phys Med Rehabil* 1973: 54: 175-179.

Other Reading

Gresham GE, Phillips TF, Labi MLC. ADL status in stroke: relative merits of three standard indexes. *Arch Phys Med Rehabil* 1980: 61: 355-358.

Iverson IA, Silverberg NE, Steven RC, Schoening HJA. *The revised Kenny Self-Care Evaluation a numerical measure of independence.* Minneapolis, MN: Sister Kenny Institute 1973.

Schoening HA, Anderegg L, Bergstrom D, Fonda M, Steinke N, Ulrich P. Numerical scoring of self care status of patients. *Arch Phys Med Rehabil* 1965: 46: 689-697.

Schoening HA, Iverson JA. Numerical scoring of self care: a study of the Kenny Self-Care Evaluation. *Arch Phys Med Rehabil* 1968: 49: 221-229.

Stern PH, McDowell F, Miller JM, Robinson M. Effects of facilitation exercise techniques in stroke rehabilitation. *Arch Phys Med Rehabil* 1973: 51: 526-531.

## A.13.	Klein-Bell Activities of Daily Living Scale

1.	Klein RM, Bell B. *Klein-Bell Activities of Daily Living Scales* 1993.

2.	Klein RM, Bell B. Self-care skills: behavioral measurement with Klein-Bell ADL Scale. *Arch Phys Med Rehabil* 1982: 63: 335-338.

## A.14.	Level of Rehabilitation Scale (LORS-II)

1.	Carey RG, Posavac EJ. *Manual for the Level of Rehabilitation Scale II.* Park Ridge II: Lutheran General Hospital 1980.

2.	Carey RG, Posavac EJ. Program evaluation of a physical medicine and rehabilitation unit: a new approach. *Arch Phys Med Rehabil* 1978: 59: 330-337.

3.	Carey RG, Posavac EJ. Rehabilitation program evaluation using a revised level of rehabilitation scale. *Arch Phys Med Rehabil* 1982: 63: 367-370.

4. Posavac EJ, Carey RG. Using a level of function scales (LORS-II) to evaluate the success of an inpatient rehabilitation program. *Rehabilitation Nursing.* 1982: 717-719.

5. Carey R, Seibert J, Posarac E. Who makes the most progress in inpatient rehabilitation? An analysis of functional gain. *Arch Phys Med Rehabil* 1988: 69 (5): 337-343.

A.15. The PULSES Profile

1. Moskowitz RW, McCann CB. Classification of disability in the chronically ill and aging. *J Chronic Dis* 1957: 5: 342-346.

2. Granger CV, Greer DS. Functional status measurement and medical rehabilitation outcomes. *Arch Phys Med Rehabil* 1976: 57: 103-109.

3. Granger CV, Albrecht GL, Hamilton BB. Outcome of comprehensive medical rehabilitation: measurement by PULSES profile and the Barthel Index. *Arch Phys Med Rehabil* 1979: 60: 145-154.

Other Reading

Granger CV, Greer DS, Liset E, Coulombe J, O'Brien E. Measurement of outcomes of care for stroke patients. *Stroke* 1975: 6: 34-41.

Granger CV, Gresham GE. Functional assessment utilization: the long-range evaluation system (LRES). In: Granger CV, Gresham GE, eds. *Functional Assessment in Rehabilitation Medicine.* Baltimore: Williams and Wilkins 1984.

Granger CV, Sherwood CC, Greer DS. Functional status measures in a comprehensive stroke care program. *Arch Phys Med Rehabil* 1977: 58: 555-561.

Mattison PG, Aitken RCB, Prescott RJ. Rehabilitation status - the relationship between the Edinburgh Rehabilitation Status Scale (ERSS), Barthel Index, and PULSES profile. *Int Disabil Stud* 1991: 13 (1): 9-11

Moskowitz E., Fuhn ER, Peters ME, Kearley AS. Aged infirm residents in a custodial institution. *Journal of the American Medical Association* 1959: 169 (17): 2009-2012.

Moskowitz E., Goldman JJ, Randall EH. A controlled study of the rehabilitation potential of nursing home residents. *New York State Medical Journal* 1960: 60: 1439-1444.

Moskowitz E., Lightbody FEH, Freitag NS. Long-term follow-up of the post-stroke patient. *Arch Phys Med Rehabil* 1972: 53: 167-172.

Moskowitz RW. PULSES profile in retrospect. *Arch Phys Med Rehabil* 1985: 66: 647-648.

Reynolds FW, Abramson M, Young A. The rehabilitation potential of patients in chronic diseases institutions. *J Chronic Dis* 1959: 10: 152-159.

A.16.   Rivermead Motor Assessment (RMA)

1.   Lincoln N, Leadbitter D. Assessment of motor function in stroke patients. *Phys Ther* 1979: 65 (2): 48-51.

2.   Endres M, Nyary I, Banhidi M, Deak G. Stroke rehabilitation: a method and evaluation. *Inter J Rehabil Res* 1990: 13: 225-236.

3.   Collen FM, Wade DT, Bradshaw CM. Mobility after stroke: reliability of measures of impairment and disability. *Int Disabil Stud* 1990: 12: 6-9.

4.   Collen FM, Wade DT, Robb GF, Bradshaw CM. The Rivermead Mobility Index: a further development of the Rivermead Motor Assessment. *Int Disabil Stud* 1991: 13: 50-54.

5.   Sackley CM, Lincoln NB. The verbal administration of the gross function scale of the Rivermead Motor Assessment. *Clinical Rehabilitation* 1990: 4: 301-303.

A.17.   Rivermead ADL Assessment

1.   Whiting S, Lincoln N. An ADL assessment for stroke patients. *British Journal of Occupational Therapy.* 1980: 43: 44-46.

2.   Lincoln N, Edmans JA. A re-validation of the Rivermead ADL scale for elderly patients with stroke. *Age and Aging* 1990: 19: 19-24.

A.18.   The Functional Autonomy Measurement System (SMAF)

1.   Hébert R, Carrier R, Bilodeau A. Elaboration d'un instrument de mesure des handicaps: Le système de mesure de l'autonomie fonctionelle (S.M.A.F). In: Montréal: Tilquin C, ed. *Editions Sciences des Systèmes* 1980.

2.   Hébert R. L'évaluation de l'autonomie fonctionelle des personnes agées. *Canadian Physician* 1982: 28: 754-762.

3. Hébert R, Bilodeau A. Profil d'autonomie fonctionnelle des personnes agées hebergées en institution.Le fonctionnement individuel et social de la personne agées. *Cahier de l'ACFAS* 1986: 46.

4. Imie PC, Eppinghaus CE, Boughton AC. Efficacy of non-bivalved and bivalved serial casting on head injured patients in intensive care. *Phys Ther* 1986: 66: 748.

5. Hébert R, Bilodeau A, Carrier R. Le système de mesure de l'autonomie fonctionelle: étude de validation. In: Van Eimeren W, Englebrecht R, Flagle CD, eds. *Third International Conference on System Science in Health Care*. Berlin: Springer Verlag 1984: 245-248.

A.19. PECS: Patient Evaluation Conference System (PECS)

1. Harvey RF, Jellinek HM. *TW3 Medical Resources Group*. University of Wisconsin-Madison 1993.

2. Harvey RF, Jellinek HM. Functional performance assessment: a program approach. *Arch Phys Med Rehabil* 1981: 62: 456-461.

3. Harvey RF, Jellinek HM. Patient profiles: Utilization in functional performance assessment. *Arch Phys Med Rehabil* 1983: 64: 268-271.

4. Korner-Bitensky N, Mayo N, Cabot R, Becker R, Coopersmith H. Motor and functional recovery after stroke: accuracy of physical therapists' predictions. *Arch Phys Med Rehabil* 1989: 70: 95-99.

5. Jellinek HM, Torkelson RM, Harvey RF. Functional abilities and distress levels in brain injured patients at long term follow-up. *Arch Phys Med Rehabil* 1982: 63: 160-162.

Other Reading

Sinyor D, Amato P, Kaloupek DG, Becker R, Goldenberg M, Coopersmith H. Post-stroke depression: Relationships to functional impairment, coping strategies, and rehabilitation outcome. *Stroke* 1986: 17: 1102-1107.

A.20. The Canadian Neurological Scale (CNS)

1. Coté R, Battista RN, Wolfson C, Boucher J. The Canadian Neurological Scale: validation and reliability assessment. *Neurology* 1989: 39 (5): 638-643.

2. Coté R, Hachinski VC, Shurvell BL, Norris JW, Wolfson C. The Canadian Neurological Scale: A preliminary study in acute stroke. *Stroke* 1986: 17 (4): 731-737.

A.21. Clinical Outcome Variable Scale (COVS)

1. Harvey RF, Jellinek HM. *TW3 Medical Resources Group.* University of Wisconsin-Madison 1993.

2. Seaby L, Torrance G. Reliability of a physiotherapy functional assessment used in a rehabilitation setting. *Physiother Can* 1989: 41 (5): 264-271.

REFERENCES FOR B. BACK AND/OR PAIN MEASURES

B.1. Visual Analogue Scale (VAS)

1. Dixon JS, Bird HA. Reproducibility along a 10 cm. vertical visual analogue scale. *Annals of the Rheumatic Diseases* 1981: 40 (1): 87-9.

2. Scott J, Huskisson EC. Vertical or horizontal visual analogue scales. *Annals of the Rheumatic Diseases* 1979: 38: 560.

3. Downie WW, Leatham PA, Rhind VM. Studies with pain rating scales. *Annals of the Rheumatic Diseases* 1978: 37: 378-381.

4. Wilkie D, Lovejoy N, Dodd M, Tesler M. Cancer pain intensity measurement: concurrent validity of three tools - finger dynameter, pain intensity number scale, visual analogue scale. *Hospice Journal* 1990: 6 (1): 1-13.

5. Langley GB, Sheppeard H. The visual analogue scale: Its use in pain measurement. *Rheumatology International.* 1985: 5: 145-148.

6. Carlsson AM. Assessment of chronic pain Part I: Aspects of the reliability and validity of the visual analogue scale. *Pain* 1983: 16: 87-101.

Other Reading

McGuire DB. The measurement of clinical pain. *Nurs Res* 1984: 33 (3): 152-156.

B.2.   Numeric Pain Rating Scale (NPRS)

1.   Jensen MP, Karoly P, Braver S. The measurement of clinical pain intensity: a comparison of six methods. *Pain* 1986: 27: 117-126.

2.   Downie WW, Leatham PA, Rhind VM. Studies with pain rating scales. *Annals of the Rheumatic Diseases* 1978: 37: 378-381.

3.   Wilkie D, Lovejoy N, Dodd M, Tesler M. Cancer pain intensity measurement: concurrent validity of three tools - finger dynameter, pain intensity number scale, visual analogue scale. *Hospice Journal* 1990: 6 (1): 1-13.

4.   McGuire DB. The measurement of clinical pain. *Nurs Res* 1984: 33 (3): 152-156.

B.3.   Pain Drawing

1.   Ransford AO, Cairns D, Mooney V. The pain drawing as an aid to the psychologic evaluation of patients with low-back pain. *Spine* 1976: 1 (2): 127-134.

2.   Schwartz DP, DeGood DE. Global appropriateness of pain drawings: Blind ratings predict patterns of psychological distress and litigation status. *Pain* 1984: 19: 383-388.

3.   Margolis RB, Tait RC, Krause SJ. A rating system for the use with patient pain drawings. *Pain* 1986: 24: 57-65.

4.   Margolis RB, Chibnall JT, Tait RC. Test-retest reliability of the pain drawing instrument. *Pain* 1988: 33: 49-51.

5.   Dzioba RB, Doxey NC. A prospective investigation and psychologic predictors of outcome of first lumbar surgery following industrial injury. *Spine* 1984: 9 (6): 614-623.

6.   Taylor WP, Stern WR, Kubiszyn TW. Predicting patients' perceptions of response to treatment for low-back pain. *Spine* 1984: 9 (3): 313-316.

7.   Greenough CG, Fraser RD. Comparison of eight psychometric instruments in unselected patients with back pain. *Spine* 1991: 16 (9): 1068-1074.

8. Von Baeyer CL, Bergstrom KJ, Brodwin MG, Brodwin SK. Invalid use of pain drawings in psychological screening of back pain patients. *Pain* 1983: 16: 103-10

Other Reading

Hildebrandt J, Franz CE, Choroba-Mehnen B, Temme M. The use of pain drawings in screening for psychological involvement in complaints of low-back pain. *Spine* 1988: 13 (6): 681-685.

Mooney V, Cairns D, Robertson J. A system for evaluating and treating chronic back disability. *The Western Journal of Medicine* 1976: 124 (5): 370-376.

B.4.   Sickness Impact Profile (SIP)

1. Bergner M, Bobbitt RA, Carter WB, Gilson BS. The sickness impact profile: Development and final revision of a health status measure. *Med Care* 1981: 19 (8): 787-805.

2. Bergner M, Bobbitt RA, Kressel S, Pollard WE, Gilson BS, Morris JR. The sickness impact profile: Conceptual formulation and methodology for the development of a health status measure. *International Journal of Health Services* 1976: 6 (3): 393-415.

3. Bergner M, Bobbitt RA, Pollard WE, Martin DP, Gilson BS. The sickness impact profile: Validation of a health measure. *Medical Care* 1976: 14 (1): 57-67.

4. Deyo RA. Measuring the functional status of patients with low back pain. *Arch Phys Med Rehabil* 1988: 69: 1044-1053.

5. Deyo RA. Comparative validity of the sickness impact profile and shorter scales for functional assessment on low-back pain. *Spine* 1986: 11 (9): 951-954.

6. Deyo RA. Pitfalls in measuring the health status of Mexican Americans: Comparative validity of the English and Spanish Sickness Impact Profile. *Health Service Research* 1976: 11: 516-528.

7. Deyo RA, Diehl AK. Measuring physical and psychosocial function in patients with low-back pain. *Spine* 1983: 8 (6): 635-642.

8. Follick MJ, Smith TW, Ahern DK. The sickness impact profile: a global measure of disability in chronic low back pain. *Pain* 1985: 21: 67-76.

9. Pollard WE, Bobbitt RA, Bergner M, Martin DP, Gilson BS. The sickness impact profile: Reliability of a health status measure. *Medical Care* 1976: 14 (2): 146-155.

B.5. Disability Questionnaire (DQ)

1. Roland M, Morris R. A study of the natural history of back pain Part 1: Development of a reliable and sensitive measure of disability in low-back pain. *Spine* 1983: 8 (2): 141-144.

2. Roland M, Morris R. A study of the natural history of back pain Part 2: Development of guidelines for trials of treatment in primary care. *Spine* 1983: 8 (2): 145-150.

3. Deyo RA. Measuring the functional status of patients with low back pain. *Arch Phys Med Rehabil* 1988: 69: 1044-1053.

4. Deyo RA. Comparative validity of the sickness impact profile and shorter scales for functional assessment on low-back pain. *Spine* 1986: 11 (9): 951-954.

B.6. Oswestry Low Back Pain Disability Questionnaire

1. Fairbanks JCT, Davies JB, Couper J, O'Brien JP. The Oswestry low-back pain disability questionaire. *Physiotherapy* 1980: 66 (8): 271-273.

Other Reading

Mayer T, Gatchel RJ. *Functional Restoration for Spinal Disorders: a Sports Medicine Approach.* Philadelphia: Lea and Febiger 1988.

Triano JJ, Schultz AB. Correlation of objective measure of trunk motion and muscle function with low-back disability ratings. *Spine* 1987: 12 (6): 561-565.

B.7. Partial Sit-up/Curl-up as a test of abdominal muscle strength/endurance

1. Faulkner RA, Sprigings EJ, McQuarrie A, Bell RD. A partial curl-up protocol for adults based on an analysis of two procedures. *Canadian Journal of Sport Science* 1989: 14 (3): 135-141.

2. Quinney HA, Smith DJ, Wenger HA. A field test for the assessment of abdominal muscular endurance in professional ice hockey players. *JOSPT* 1984: 6 (1): 30-33.

3. Ricci B, Marchetti M, Figura F. Biomechanics of sit-up exercises. *Med Sci Sports Exerc* 1981: 13 (1): 54-59.

4. Richardson C, Toppenberg R, Jull G. An initial evaluation of eight abdominal exercises for their ability to provide stabilization for the lumbar spine. *Australian Physiotherapy* 1990: 36 (1): 6-11.

B.8.   Sorensen Test for endurance of the back musculature

1.   Biering-Sorensen F. Physical measurements as risk indicators for low-back trouble over a one-year period. *Spine* 1984: 9 (2): 106-119.

2.   Nordin M, Kahanovitz N, Verderame R. Normal trunk muscle strength and endurance in women and the effects of exercise and electrical stimulation Part 1: Normal endurance and trunk muscle strength in 101 women. *Spine* 1987: 12 (2): 105-111.

B.9.   Pressure Biofeedback (PBF) for measuring muscular endurance of the transverse abdominal and abdominal oblique musculature

1.   Jull GA, Richardson CA. *The Muscular Protection of the Lumbar Spine.* Proceedings of National Orthopaedic Symposium, Orthopaedic Division, C.P.A.. Toronto 1992: 77-83.

2.   Richardson C, Jull G, Toppenberg R, Comerford M. Techniques for active lumbar stabilization for spinal protection: A pilot study. *Australian Physiotherapy* 1992: 38 (2): 105-112.

3.   Richardson C, Sims K. An inner range holding contraction: An objective measure of stabilizing function in an antigravity muscle. In: *Proceedings: World Confederation of Physical Therapy 11th International Congress.* World Confederation of Physical Therapy 1993.

4.   Richardson C, Toppenberg R, Jull G. An initial evaluation of eight abdominal exercises for their ability to provide stabilization for the lumbar spine. *Australian Physiotherapy* 1990: 36 (1): 6-11.

B.10.   Modified Schober method of measuring spinal mobility

1.   Macrae IF, Wright V. Measurement of back movement. *Annals of the Rheumatic Diseases* 1969: 28: 584-589.

2.   Moll JM, Wright V. Normal range of spinal mobility. An objective clinical study. *Annals of the Rheumatic Diseases* 1971: 30: 381-386.

3.   Williams R, Binkley J, Bloch R. Reliability of the modified-modified Schober and double inclinometer methods for measuring lumbar flexion and extension. *Phys Ther* 1993: 73 (1): 26-37.

4.   Miller MH, Lee P, Smythe HA, Goldsmith C. Measurement of spinal mobility in the sagittal plane: new skin contraction technique compared with established methods. *Journal of Rheumatology* 1984: 11 (4): 507-511.

5.   Gill K, Krag MH, Johnson GB, Haugh LD, Pope MH. Repeatability of four clinical methods for assessment of lumbar spinal motion. *Spine* 1988: 13 (1): 50-53.

6.   Portek I, Pearcy MJ, Reader GP, Mowat AG. Correlation between radiographic and clinical measurement of lumbar spine movement. *British Journal of Rheumatology* 1983: 22: 197-205.

7.   Reynolds PMG. Measurement of spinal mobility: A comparison of three methods. *Rheumatol Rehabil* 1975: 14: 180-185.

8.   Beattie P, Rothstein JM, Lamb RL. Reliability of the attraction method for measuring lumbar spine backward bending. *Phys Ther* 1987: 67 (3): 364-369.

9.   Pile KD, Laurent MR, Salmond CE, Best BJ, Pyle EA, Moloney RO. Clinical assessment of ankylosing spondylitis: a study of observer variation in spinal measurements. *British Journal of Rheumatology* 1991: 30: 29-34.

10.   Miller SA, Mayer T, Cox R, Gatchel RJ. Reliability problems associated with the modified Schober technique for true lumbar flexion measurement. *Spine* 1992: (17) 3: 345-348.

B.11.   Leighton Flexometer for measuring spinal mobility

1.   Leighton JR. The Leighton flexometer and flexibility test. *The Journal of the Association for Physical and Mental Rehabilitation.* 1958: 20: 127-130.

Other Reading

Harris ML. A factor analytic study of flexibility. *Research Quarterly* 1969: 40 (1): 62-70.

MacDougall JD, Wenger HA, Green HJ. *Physiological Testing of the High-Performance Athlete.* 2nd ed. Champaign Illinois: Human Kinetics Books 1991.

Munroe RA, Romance TJ. Use of the Leighton Flexometer in the development of a short flexibility test battery. *American Correctional Therapy Journal* 1975: 29 (1): 22-25.

B.12. Inclinometer method of measuring spinal mobility

1. Loebl WY. Measurement of spinal posture and range of spinal movement. *Annals of Physical Medicine* 1967: 9: 104-110.

2. Miller MH, Lee P, Smythe HA, Goldsmith C. Measurment of spinal mobility in the sagittal plane: new skin contraction technique compared with established methods. *Journal of Rheumatology* 1984: 11 (4): 507-511.

3. Reynolds PMG. Measurement of spinal mobility: A comparison of three methods. *Rheumatol Rehabil* 1975: 14: 180-185.

4. Keeley J, Mayer TG, Cox R, Gatchel RJ, Smith J, Mooney V. Quantification of lumbar function Part 5: Reliability of range of motion measures in the sagittal plane and in vivo torso rotation measurement technique. *Spine* 1986: 11 (1):31-35.

5. Boline PD, Keating JC, Haas M, Anderson AV. *Interexaminer reliability and discriminant validity of inclinometric measurement of lumbar rotation in chronic low-back pain patients and subjects without low-back pain* 1993.

6. Gill K, Krag MH, Johnson GB, Haugh LD, Pope MH. Repeatability of four clinical methods for assessment of lumbar spinal motion. *Spine* 1988;13 (1):50-53.

7. Williams R, Binkley J, Bloch R. Reliability of the modified-modified Schober and double inclinometer methods for measuring lumbar flexion and extension. *Phys Ther* 1993: 73 (1): 26-37.

8. Mayer TG, Tencer AF, Kristofferson S, Mooney V. Use of non-invasive techniques for quantification of spinal range of motion in normal subjects and chronic low-back dysfunction patients. *Spine* 1984: 9 (6): 588-595.

9. Newton M, Waddell G. Reliability and validity of clinical measurement of the lumbar spine in patients with chronic low-back pain. *Physiotherapy* 1991;77 (12): 796-800.

10. Portek I, Pearcy MJ, Reader GP, Mowat AG. Correlation between radiographic and clinical measurement of lumbar spine movement. *British Journal of Rheumatology* 1983: 22: 197-205.

B.13. Lifting Dynamometers

1.   Mayer T, Gatchel RJ. *Functional Restoration for Spinal Disorders: a Sports Medicine Approach*. Philadelphia: Lea and Febiger 1988.

2.   Kishino ND, Mayer TG, Gatchel RJ. Quantification of lumbar function Part 4: Isometric and isokinetic lifting stimulation in normal subjects and low back dysfunction patients. *Spine* 1985: 10 (10): 921-927.

3.   Hazard RG, Fenwick J, Kalish S. Functional restoration with behavioural support: A one year prospective study with chronic low-back pain. *Spine* 1989: 14 (2): 157-161.

B.14. Isokinetic Dynamometers

1.   Hasue M, Masatoshi F, Kikuchi S. A new method of quantitative measurement of abdominal and back muscle strength. *Spine* 1980: 2 (5): 143-147.

2.   Mayer TG, Smith SS, Kondraske G, Gatchell RJ, Carmeichael TW, Mooney V. Quantification of lumbar function Part 3: Preliminary data on isokinetic torso rotation testing with myoelectric spectral analysis in normal and low-back pain subjects. *Spine* 1985: 10 (10): 912-920.

3.   Suzuki N, Endo S. A quantative study of trunk muscle strength and fatigability in the low-back syndrome. *Spine* 1983: 8 (1): 69-74.

Other Reading

Hazard RG, Reid S, Fenwick J, Reeves V. Isokinetic trunk and lifting strength measurements: Variability as an indicator of effort. *Spine* 1988: 13 (1): 54-57.

Mayer TG, Gatchell RJ, Kishino N. Objective assessment of spine function following industrial injury: A prospective study with comparison group and one-year follow-up. *Spine* 1985: 10 (6): 482-493.

Mayer TG, Smith SS, Keeley J, Mooney V. Quantification of lumbar function Part 2: Sagittal plane trunk strength in chronic low-back pain patients. *Spine* 1985: 10 (8): 764-772.

Smith SS, Mayer TG, Gatchell RJ, Becker TJ. Quantification of lumbar function Part 1: Isometric and multi-speed isokinetic trunk strength measures in sagittal and axial planes in normal subjects. *Spine* 1985: 10 (8): 757-763.

Timm KE, Malone TR. Back Injuries and Rehabilitation Sports Injury Managment: A Quarterly Series. *Back Injuries and Rehabilitation Sports Injury Management* 1989: 2 (3): 50-56.

REFERENCES FOR C. CARDIOPULMONARY MEASURES

C.1. Heart Rate

1. Hurst JW, Shlant RC. *The Heart.* 7th ed. Toronto: McGraw Hill Information Services Company 1990.

2. Astrand PO, Rodahl K. *Textbook of Work Physiology: Physiological Bases of Exercise.* 2nd ed. New York: McGraw-Hill 1977.

3. Cotton FS, Dill DB. On the relation between the heart rate during exercise and that of immediate post-exercise period. *American Journal of Physiology* 1935: 111: 554-556.

4. Pollock ML, Broida J. Kendrick Z. Validity of the palpation technique of heart rate determination and its estimation of training heart rate. *Res Q Am Assoc Health Phys Ed.* 1972: 43: 77-81.

5. McArdle WD, Zwiren L, Magel JR. Validity of the post exercise heart rate as a means of estimating heart rate during work of varying intensities. *Res Q Am Assoc Health Phys Ed.* 1969: 40: 523-509.

6. Rothstein JM. *Measurement in Physical Therapy.* New York: Churchill Livingstone 1985.

7. Sedlock DA, Knowlton RG, Fitzgerald PI, Tahamont MV, Schneider DA. Accuracy of subject-palpated carotid pulse after exercise. *Phys Sports Med* 1983: 11: 106-116.

C.2. Blood Pressure

1. Eilertsen E, Humerfelt S. The observer variation in the measurement of arterial blood pressure. *Acta Med Scand* 1968: 184: 145-157.

2. Fagan TC, Conrad KA, Mayshar PV, Mackie MJ, Hagaman RM. Single versus triplicate measurements of blood pressure and heart rate. *Hypertens* 1988: 11: 282-284.

3. Roberts LN. A comparison of direct and indirect blood pressure determinations. *Circ* 1953: 8: 232.

4. Holland WW, Humerfelt S. Measurements of blood pressure: comparison of intraarterial and cuff values. *Br Med J.* 1964: 2: 1241-1243.

5.   Van Bergen FH, Weatherhead DS, Treloar AE, Dobkin AB, Buckley JJ. Comparison of indirect and direct methods of measuring arterial blood pressure. *Circ* 1954: 10: 481-490.

6.   Mellerowicz H, Smodlaka VN. *Ergometry and Basics of Medical Exercise Testing*. Baltimore: Urban and Svhwarzenberg 1981.

7.   Stolt M. Reliability of auscultatory method of arterial blood pressure. *Hypertens* 1990: 3 (9): 697-703.

8.   Karvonen MJ, Telivuo LJ, Jarvinen JK . Sphygmomanometer cuff size and the accuracy of indirect measurement of blood pressure. *Am J Cardiol* 1964: 13: 688-693.

9.   Neilsen PE, Janniche H. The accuracy of auscultatory measurement of arm blood pressure in very obese subjects. *Acta Med Scand* 1974: 195: 403-409.

10.   Geddes LA, Whistler SJ. The error in indirect blood pressure measurement with the incorrect size of cuff. *Am Heart J* 1978: 96: 4-8.

11.   Neilsen PE et al. Accuracy of auscultatory blood pressure measurements in hypertensive and obese subjects. *Hypertens* 1983: 5: 122-127.

12.   Burke MJ. Sphygmomanometers in hospital and family practice: problems and recommendations. *Br Med J.* 1982: 285: 469-471.

Other Reading

Frohlich ED. Recommendations for human blood pressure determination by sphygmomanometers. Report of a special task force appointed by the steering committee, American Heart Association. *Hypertens* 1988: 11 (2): 210A-222A.

Hurst JW, Shlant RC. *The Heart*. 7th ed. Toronto: McGraw Hill Information Services Company 1990.

Simpson JA, Jamieson G, Dickhaus DW, Grover RF. Effect of size of cuff bladder on accuracy of measurement of indirect blood pressure. *Am Heart J.* 1965: 70: 208-215.

C.3.   Respiratory Rate

1.   Simoes EAF, et al. Respiratory rate: measurement of variability over time and accuracy at different counting periods. *Arch Dis Childhood* 1991: 66 (10): 1199-1203.

C.4. Percussion

1. Parrino TA. The art and science of percussion. *Hosp Prac.* 1987: 22: 25-36.

2. Smyllie HC, et al. Observer agreement in physical signs of the respiratory system. *Lancet* 1965: 289: 412-413.

3. Godfrey S, et al. Repeatability of physical signs in airways obstruction. *Thorax* 1969: 24: 4-9.

4. Spiteri MA, et al. Reliability of eliciting physical signs in examination of the chest. *Lancet* 1988: 1: 873-875.

5. Guarino JR. Auscultatory percussion of the chest. *Lancet* 1980: 1: 1332-1334.

6. Bourke S, et al. Percussion of the chest re-visited: a comparison of the diagnostic value of auscultatory and conventional chest percussion. *Ir J Med Sci.* 1989: 158: 82-84.

7. Ogilvie C. *Chamberlain's Symptoms and Signs in Clinical Medicine.* 10th ed. Bristol, England: Wright and Sons Limited 1980.

C.5. Auscultation of Lung Sounds

1. Mikami R, et al. International symposium of lung sounds. Synopsis of proceedings. *Chest* 1987: 92 (2): 342-345.

2. Schilling RSF, et al. Disagreement between observers in an epidemiological study of respiratory disease. *Br Med J.* 1955 Jan 8: 65-68.

3. Smyllie HC, et al. Observer agreement in physical signs of the respiratory system. *Lancet* 1965: 289: 412-413.

4. Godfrey S, et al. Repeatability of physical signs in airways obstruction. *Thorax* 1969: 4: 4-9.

5. Pasterkamp H, et al. Nomenclature used by health care professionals to describe breath sounds in asthma. *Chest* 1993: 92 (2): 346-352.

6. Spiteri MA, et al. Reliability of eliciting physical signs in examination of the chest. *Lancet* 1988: 1: 873-875.

7. Aweida D, Kelsey CJ. Accuracy and reliability of physical therapists in auscultating tape-recorded lung sounds. *Physiother Can* 1990: 42 (6): 279-282.

8. Brooks D, et al. Accuracy and reliability of specialized physical therapists in auscultating tape recorded lungs sounds. *Physiother Can* 1993: 45 (1): 21-24.

Other Reading

ACCP-ATS Joint Committee on Pulmonary Nomenclature. Pulmonary terms and symbols. *Chest* 1975: 67: 5-10.

Report of the ATS-ACCP Ad Hoc Subcommittee on Pulmonary Nomenclature. *American Thoracic Society News* 1977: 26-34.

C.6. Chronic Respiratory Disease Questionnaire

1. Guyatt G, Berman LB, Townsend M, Pugsley SO, Chambers LW. A measure of quality of life for clinical trials in chronic lung disease. *Thorax* 1987: 42: 773-778.

2. Guyatt GH, et al. Measuring functional status in chronic lung disease: conclusions from a randomized control trial. *Respir Med.* 1989: 83 (4): 293-297.

3. Guyatt GH, et al. Should study subjects see their previous responses: data from a randomized control trial. *J Clinical Epidemiol.* 1989: 42 (9): 913-920.

C.7. Visual Analogue Scale for Dyspnea

1. Aitken RCB. Measurement of feelings using visual analogue scales. *Proc R Soc Med* 1969: 62: 989-993.

2. Mahler DA. *Dyspnea.* Mt Kisco, New York: Futura Publishing Company, Inc. 1990.

3. Muza SR. Comparison of scales used to quantitate the sense of effort to breathe in patients with chronic obstructive pulmonary disease. *Am Rev Respir Dis.* 1990: 141: 909-913.

4. Gift AG. Validation of a vertical visual analogue scale as a measure of clinical dyspnea. *Rehabilitation Nursing.* 1989: 14: 323-325.

5. Gift AG, Cahill A. Psychophysiologic aspects of dyspnea in COPD: a pilot study. *Heart Lung* 1990: 19 (3): 252-257.

6. Wilson RC, Jones PW. A comparison of the visual analogue scale and the modified Borg scale for the measurement of dyspnea during exercise. *Clin Sci*. 1989: 76: 277-282.

C.8. Six-Minute Walking Test

1. Cooper KH. A means of assessing maximal oxygen intake. *JAMA* 1968: 203 (3): 135-138.

2. Cooper KH. *The new Aerobics*. New York: Evans and Company Inc. 1970.

3. McGavin CR, Gupta SP, McHardy GJ. Twelve minute walking test for assessing disability in chronic bronchitis. *Br Med J*. 1976: 1: 822-823.

4. McGavin CR. Physical rehabilitation for the chronic bronchitic: results of a controlled trial of exercises in the home. *Thorax* 1977: 32: 307-311.

5. Butland RJA, Pang J, Gross ER, Woodcock AA, Geddes DM. Two-, six-, and 12-minute walking tests in respiratory disease. *Br Med J* 1982: 284: 1607-1608.

6. Guyatt GH, Pugsley SO, Sullivan MJ, et al. Effect of encouragement on walking test performance. *Thorax* 1984: 39: 818-822.

7. Guyatt GH, Sullivan MJ, Thompson PJ, et al. The 6-minute walk: a new measure of exercise capacity in patients with chronic heart failure. *Can Med Assoc* 1985: 132: 919-923.

8. Guyatt GH, Thompson PJ, Berman LB, et al. How should we measure function in patients with chronic heart and lung disease. *J Chron Dis*. 1985: 38 (6): 517-524.

9. Mungall IPF, Hainsworth R. Assessment of respiratory function in patients with chronic obstructive airways disease. *Thorax* 1979: 34: 254-258.

10. McGavin CR. Dyspnoea, disability, and distance walked: comparison of estimates of exercise performance in respiratory disease. *Br Med J*. 1978: 2: 241-243.

11. Dekhuyzen PNR. Twelve minute walking test in a group of Dutch patients with chronic obstructive pulmonary diseases: relationship with functional capacity. *Eur J Respir Dis*. 1986: 69 (Suppl. 146): 259-264.

12.   ZuWallack RL. Predictors of improvement in the 12-minute walking distance following a six week outpatient pulmonary rehabilitation program. *Chest* 1991: 99 (4): 805-808.

13.   Guyatt GH, Townsend M, Keller J, Singer J, Nogradi S. Measuring functional status in chronic lung disease: conclusions from a randomized control trial. *Resp Med.* 1989: 83: 293-297.

14.   Beaumount A. A self paced treadmill walking test for breathless patients. *Thorax* 1985: 40: 459-464.

15.   Swerts PMJ. Comparison of corridor and treadmill walking in patients with severe chronic obstructive pulmonary disease. *Phys Ther* 1990: 70 (7): 439-442.

16.   Swinburnd CR, Wakefield JM, Jones PW. Performance, ventilation and oxygen consumption in three different types of exercise test in patients with chronic obstructive lung disease. Thorax 1985: 40 (8): 581-586.

C.9.   Self-Paced Walking Test to predict VO_2 max

1.   Astrand PO, Rodahl K. *Textbook of Work Physiology: Physiological Bases of Exercise*. 2nd ed. New York: McGraw-Hill 1977.

2.   Bassey EJ, Fenton PH, MacDonald IC. Self-paced walking as a method for exercise testing in elderly and young men. *Clinical Science and Molecular Medicine* 1976: 51: 609-612.

3.   Martin PE, Rothstein DE, Larish DD. Effects of age and physical activity status on speed-aerobic demand relationships of walking. *Journal of Applied Physiology* 1993: 73 (1): 200-206.

Other Reading

Cunningham DA, Rechnitzer PA, Donner AP. Exercise training and the speed of self-selected walking pace in men at retirement. *Canadian Journal on Aging* 1986: 5 (1): 19-25.

Francis K. The use of the walk test for the development of exercise guidelines. *Computerized Biological Medicine* 1991: 21 (3): 111-120.

McBeath AA, Bahrke MS, Balke B. Walking efficiency before and after total hip replacement as determined by oxygen consumption. *Journal of Bone and Joint Surgery* 1980: 62A (5): 807-810.

C.10. Vital Capacity

1. American Thoracic Society . Standardization of Spirometry - 1987 Update. *Am Rev Respir Dis*. 1987: 136: 1285-1298.

2. American Thoracic Society . Lung Function Testing: Selection of reference values and interpretive strategies. *Am Rev Respir Dis*. 1991: 144: 1202-1218.

3. Knudson RJ, Burrows B. Early detection of obstructive lung disease. *Med Clin Am* 1973: 3: 681-690.

4. Thurlbeck WM. Small airways: physiology meets pathology. *N Engl J Med* 1978: 298: 1310-1311.

5. Nickerson BJ. Within subject variability and percent change for significance of spirometry in normal subjects and patients with cystic fibrosis. *Am Rev Respir Dis*. 1980: 122: 859-866.

6. Cosio M, Ghezzo IT, Hogg JC, et al. The relations between structural changes in small airways and pulmonary function tests. *N Engl J Med* 1978: 298: 1277-1281.

7. Hogg JC, MacKlem PT, Thurlbeck WM. Site and nature of airway obstruction in chronic lung disease. *N Engl J Med* 1968: 278: 1355-1360.

Other Reading

Clausen JL (Ed.). *Pulmonary Function Testing Guidelines and Controversies*. Toronto: Academic Press 1982.

Cochrane GM et al. Intrasubject variability of maximum expiratory flow volume curve. *Thorax* 1977: 32: 171-176.

Loss RW, Hall WJ, Speers DM. Evaluation of early airway disease in smokers: cost effectiveness of pulmonary function testing. *Am J Med Sci* 1979: 278: 27-37.

Love RG, Attfield MD, Isles KD. Reproducibility of pulmonary function tests under laboratory and field conditions. *Br J Int Med*. 1980: 37: 63-69.

MacDonald JB, Cole TJ. The flow-volume loop: reproducibility of air and helium based tests in normal subjects. *Thorax* 1980: 35: 64-69.

Marco M, Minette A. Lung function changes in smokers with normal conventional spirometry. *Am Rev Respir Dis*. 1976: 114: 723-738.

Mungall IPF, Hainsworth R. Assessment of respiratory function in patients with chronic obstructive airways disease. *Thorax* 1979: 34: 254-258.

Rothstein JM. *Measurement in Physical Therapy*. New York: Churchill Livingstone 1985.

C.11. Peak Expiratory Flow Rate (PEFR)

1. American Thoracic Society . Standardization of Spirometry - 1987 Update. *Am Rev Respir Dis*. 1987: 136: 1285-1298.

2. American Thoracic Society . Lung Function Testing: Selection of reference values and interpretive strategies. *Am Rev Respir Dis*. 1991: 144: 1202.

3. Clausen JL et al. *Pulmonary Function Testing Guidelines and Controversies*. Toronto: Academic Press 1982.

4. Hetzel MR, Clark TJH. Comparison of normal and asthmatic circadian rhythms in peak expiratory flow rate. *Thorax* 1980: 35: 732-738.

5. Clark TJM, Hetzel MR. Diurnal variation of asthma. *Br J Dis Chest* 1977: 71: 87-92.

6. Bagg LR, Hughes DT. Diurnal variation in peak expiratory flow in asthmatics. *Eur J Respir Dis*. 1980: 61: 298-302.

7. Afschrift M et al. Maximal expiratory and inspiratory flow in patients with chronic obstructive pulmonary disease: influence of bronchodilation. *Am Rev Respir Dis*. 1969: 100: 147-152.

8. Tashkin DP. The UCLA population studies of chronic obstructive respiratory disease: II. Determination of reliability and estimation of sensitivity and specificity. *Environ Res*. 1979: 20: 403-424.

9. Stanescu D, Veriter C, Van Leeputten R, Brasseur L. Constancy of effort and variability of maximum expiratory flow rates. *Chest* 1979: 76: 59-63.

10. Cosio M, Ghezzo H, Hogg JC, et al. The relations between structural changes in small airways and pulmonary function tests. *N Engl J Med* 1978: 298: 1277.

11. Thurlbeck WM. Small airways: physiology meets pathology. *N Engl J Med* 1978; 298: 1310-1311.

Other Reading

Rothstein JM. *Measurement in Physical Therapy*. New York: Churchill Livingstone 1985.

C.12. Maximum Inspiratory and Expiratory Pressures (MIP's/MEP's or MIF/MEF or PImax/PEmax

1. Rohrer F. Der Zusammenhand, Jer Atemkräfte und ihre Abhängigkeit vorm Dehnungszustand der Atmungsorgane.*Pfluegers Arch Ges Physiol* 1916: 165: 419-444.

2. Rahn H, Otis AB, Chadwick LE, Fenn WO. The pressure-volume diagram of the thorax and lung. *American Journal of Physiology* 1946: 146: 161-178.

3. Clausen JL (Ed.). *Pulmonary Function Testing Guidelines and Controversies*. Toronto: Academic Press 1982.

4. Black LF, Hyatt RE. Maximal respiratory pressures: normal values and relationship to age and sex. *Am Rev Respir Dis.* 1969: 99: 696-702.

5. Marini JJ, et al. Estimation of inspiratory muscle strength in mechanically ventilated patients: the measurement of maximum inspiratory pressure. *J Crit Care.* 1986; 1 (1):32-38.

6. Rubenstein I. Assessment of maximum expiratory pressure in health adults. *Journal of Applied Physiology* 1988: 64 (5): 2215-2219.

7. Smyth RJ, et al. Maximal inspiratory and expiratory pressures in adolescents: normal values. *Chest* 1984: 86: 568-572.

8. Wilson SH, et al. Predicted normal values for maximum respiratory pressures in caucasian adults and children. *Thorax* 1984: 39: 535-538.

9. Derenne JP, MacKlen PT, Roussos C, et al. The respiraory muscles: mechanics, control and pathophysiology. *Am Rev Respir Dis.* 1978: 118: 119-133.

10. Derenne JP, MacKlen PT, Roussos C, et al. The Mechanics, Control and Pathophysiology - Part III. AM Rev. Respir Dis 118(3): 581-601.

Other Reading

Leech JA et al. Respiratory pressures and function in young adults. *Am Rev Respir Dis.* 1983: 128: 17-23.

C.13. Oxygen Saturation

1. Technology Subcommittee of the Working Group on Critical Care OMH. Noninvasive blood gas monitoring: a review for use in the adult critical care unit. *Can Med Assoc* 1992: 146 (5): 703-712.

2. Clayton DG, et al. A comparison of the performance of 20 pulse oximeters under conditions of poor perfusion. *Anaesth* 1991: 46: 3-10.

3. Yelderman M, New W. Evaluation of pulse oximetry. *Anesthesiol.* 1983: 59 (4): 349-352.

4. Mengelkock LJ et al. A review of the principles of pulse oximetry and accuracy of pulse oximeter estimates during exercise. *Phys Ther* 1994: 74: 40-44.

5. Taylor MB, Whitwam JG. The accuracy of pulse oximeters. *Anaesth.* 1988: 43: 229-232.

6. Reis AL, et al. Accuracy of two ear oximeters at rest and during exercise in pulmonary patients. *Am Rev Resp Dis* 1985: 132: 685-689.

7. Servinghaus JW. History, status and future of pulse oximetry. *Adv Exp Med Biol* 1987: 220: 3-8.

8. Nickerson BG, et al. Bias and precision of pulse oximeters and arterial oximeters. *Chest* 1988: 93: 515-517.

9. Kelleher JF. Pulse oximetry. *J Clin Monit.* 1989: 5 (1): 37-62.

REFERENCES FOR D. DEVELOPMENTAL MEASURES

D.1. Alberta Infant Motor Scale (AIMS

1. Piper MC, Pinnell LE, Darrah J, Maguire T, Byrne PJ. Construction and validation of the Alberta Infant Motor Scale (AIMS). *Canadian Journal of Public Health.* 1992: 83: 46-50.

2. Piper MC, Darrah J. *Motor Assessment of the Developing Infant.* Philadelphia: WB Sanders 1994.

D.2. Bayley Scales of Infant Development (Psychomotor Scale)

1. Bayley N. *Manual for the Bayley Scales of Infant Development*. New York: Psychological Corporation 1969.

2. Werner EE, Bayley N. The reliability of Bayley's Revised Scale of mental and motor development during the first year of life. *Child Dev* 1966: 37: 39-50.

3. Siegel LS. Infant test of predictors of cognitive and language development at two years. *Child Dev* 1981: 52: 545-556.

4. Palisano RJ. Concurrent and predictive validities of the Bayley Motor Scale and the Peabody Developmental Motor Scales. *Phys Ther* 1986: 66 (11): 1714-1719.

5. Crowe TK, Deitz JC, Bennett FC. The relationship between the Bayley Scales of infant development and Preschool Gross Motor and Cognitive performance. *Am J of OT* 1987: 41 (6): 374-378.

6. Gannon DR. Relationship between 8 month performance on the Bayley Scales of infant development and 48 month intelligence and concept formation scores. *Psychol Rep* 1968: 23(3): 1199-1205.

7. Harris SR. Early detection of cerebral palsy: sensitivity and specificity of two motor assessment tools. *J Perinatol* 1987: 7 (1): 11-15.

8. Berk RA. The discriminative efficiency of the Bayley Scales of infant development. *Journal of Abnormal Child Psychology* 1979: 7: 113-11 9.

Other Reading

Campbell SK, Wilhelm IJ. Development from birth to 3 years of age of 15 children at high risk for central nervous system dysfunction; Interim report. *Phys Ther* 1985: 65 (4): 463-469.

Campbell SK, Siegel E, Parr CA, Ramsey CT. Evidence for the need to renorm the Bayley Scales of Infant Development based on the performance of the population-based sample of twelve-month old infants. *Topics in Early Childhood Special Education* 1986: 6 (2): 83-96.

Coryell J, Provost B, Wilhelm IJ, Campbell SK. Stability of Bayley Motor Scales in the first year of life. *Phys Ther* 1989: 69: 834-841.

Eipper DS, Azen SP. A comparison of two developmental instruments in evaluating children with Down's Syndrome. *Phys Ther* 1978: 58 (9): 1066-1069.

Harris SR, Thompson M, McGrew L. Motor assessment tools: their concurrent validity in evaluating children with multiple handicaps. *Arch Phys Med Rehabil* 1983: 64: 468-470.

Horner TM. Test-retest and home-clinic characteristics of the Bayley Scales of infant development in nine and fifteen-month-old infants. *Child Dev* 1980: 51: 751-758.

Nelson MN. *Bayley Developmental Assessments of Low Birthweight Infants*. New York, NY.: SP Medical and Scientific Books 1979: 301-308.

Paban M, Piper MC. Early predictors of one year neurodevelopmental outcome for "at risk" infants. *Physical and Occupational Therapy in Pediatrics* 19877 (3): 17-34.

Ramsey CT, Campbell FA, Nicholson JE. The predictive power of the Bayley Scales of Infant Development and the Stanford-Binet Test in a relatively constant environment. *Child Dev* 1973: 44: 790-795.

D.3.   Peabody Developmental Motor Scales

1.   Folio R, Fewell RR. *Peabody Developmental Motor Scales and Activity Cards*. Hingham, MA: DL.M Teaching Resources 1983.

2.   Folio R, Dubose RF. Peabody Development Motor Scale (rev. experimental ed.). *I MRID Behavioural Science Monograph* 1974: 25.

3.   Jenkins JR, Sells CJ, Brady D. Effects of developmental therapy on motor impaired children. *Physical and Occupational Therapy in Pediatrics* 1992: 2 (4): 19-28.

4.   Lydic JS, Short MA, Nelson DI. Comparison of two scales for assessing motor development in infants with Down's syndrome. *The Occupational Therapy Journal of Research* 1983: 3 (4): 213-221.

5.   Ottenbacher K, Short MA, Watson PJ. The effects of a clinically applied program of vestibular stimulation on the neuromotor performance of children with severe developmental disability. *Physical and Occupational Therapy in Pediatrics* 1981: 1: 1-11.

6.   Palisano PJ, Lydic JS. The Peabody Developmental Motor Scales: an analysis. *Physical and Occupational Therapy in Pediatrics* 1984: 4 (1): 69-75.

7.   Palisano RJ. Concurrent and predictive validities of the Bayley Motor Scale and the Peabody Developmental Motor Scales. *Phys Ther* 1986: 66 (11): 1714-1719.

8.   Palisano RJ. Use of chronological and adjusted age to compare motor development of healthy pre-term infants to full-term infants. *Dev Med Child Neurol* 1986: 28: 180-187.

9.   Shinderer KA, Richardson PPK, Atwater SW. Clincial implications of the Peabody Developmental Motor Scales : A constructive view. *Physical and Occupational Therapy in Pediatrics* 1989: 9 (2): 81-106.

10.   Stephens TE, Haley SM. Comparison of two methods for determining change in motorically handicapped children. *Physical and Occupational Therapy in Pediatrics* 1991: 11 (1): 1-17.

11.   Stokes NA, Deitz JL, Crowe TK. The Peabody developmental fine motor scale: an interrater reliability. *AJOT* 1990: 44 (4): 334-340.

D.4.   Test of Motor and Neurological Functions (TMNF)

1.   DeGangi GA, Berk RA, Valvano J. Test of motor and neurological functions in high-risk infants: preliminary findings. *Developmental and Behavioral Pediatrics* 1983: 4 (3): 182-189.

2.   Russell D, Rosenbaum P, Cadman D, Gowland C, Hardy S, Degani GA, et al. Toward a methodology of the short-term effects of neurodevelopmental treatment. *AJOT* 1983: 37: 479-484.

3.   Valvano J, DeGangi GA. Atypical posture and movement findings in high risk and preterm infants. *Physical and Occupational Therapy in Pediatrics* 1986: 6: 71-81.

D.5.   Test of Motor Impairment

1.   Stott DH, Moyes FA, Henderson SE. *Test of Motor Impairment*. Guelph, Ontario: Brook Educational Publishing Limited 1972.

D.6.   Posture and Fine Motor Assessment of Infants (PFMAI)

1.   Case-Smith J. Reliability and validity of the posture and fine motor assessment of infants. *The Occupational Therapy Journal of Research* 1989: 9 (5): 259-272.

2.   Case-Smith J. *The Posture and Fine Motor Assessment of Infants*. Department of Occupational Therapy, University of Richmond Virginia 1993 (unpublished paper).

D.7. Basic Gross Motor Assessment (BGMA)

1. Hughes JE. *Basic Gross Motor Assessment*. Golden CO., Jeanne E. Hughes 1979.

2. Hughes JE, Riley A. Basic Gross Motor Assessment: Tool for use with children having minor motor dysfunction. *Phys Ther* 1981: 61 (1): 503-511.

D.8. Bruininks-Oseretsky Test of Motor Proficiency (BOTMP)

1. Bruininks RH. *Bruininks-Oseretsky test of motor proficiency: examiner's manual*. United States of America: American Guidance Service Inc. 1978.

2. Broadhead GD, Bruininks RH. Factor structure consistency in the childhood motor performance traits on the Bruininks-Oseretsky test shortform. *Rehabitation Literature*. 1983: 44 (1-2): 13-18.

3. Krus PH, Bruininks RH. Structure of motor abilities in children. *Percept Mot Skills* 1981: 52: 119-129.

4. Verderber JMS, Payne VG. A comparison of the long and short forms of the Bruininks-Oseretsky test of motor proficiency. *Physical Activity Quarterly* 1987: 4: 51-59.

D.9. Gross Motor Function Measure (GMFM)

1. Rosenbaum P, Cadman D, Russell D, Gowland C, Hardy S, Jarvis S. Issues in measuring change in motor function in children with cerebral palsy. A special communication. *Phys Ther* 1990: 70: 125-131.

2. Russell D, Rosenbaum P, Gowland C, Hardy S, Cadman D. Validation of a gross motor measure for children with cerebral palsy. *Physiother Can* 1990: 42 (Suppl 3): 2.

3. Russell D, Rosenbaum P, Gowland C, et al. *Gross Motor Function Measure (GMFM): A measure of gross motor function in cerebral palsy*. Hamilton, Ontario: McMaster University 1990.

4. Russell D, Rosenbaum P, Cadman D, Gowland C, Hardy S, Jarvis S. The Gross Motor Function Measure: A means to evaluate the effects of physical therapy. *Dev Med Child Neurol* 1989: 31: 341-352.

D.10. Gross Motor Performance Measure (GMPM)

1. Boyce W, Gowland C, Hardy S, et al. Reliability of the gross motor performance measure of cerebral palsy. *Physiother Can* 1990: 42 (Suppl):1.

2. Boyce W, Gowland C, Hardy S, et al. Development of a quality of movement measure for children with cerebral palsy. *Phys Ther* 1991: 71: 820-832.

3. Boyce W, Gowland C, Rosenbaum P, et al. Gross Motor Performance Measure for children with cerebral palsy: study design and preliminary findings. *Canadian Journal of Public Health* 1992: 83 Supplement: s34-s40.

4. Boyce W, Gowland C, Russell D, et al. Consensus methodology in the development and content validation of a gross motor performance measure. *Physiother Can* 1993: 45 (2): 94-100.

5. Berg KO, Williams JI, Wood-Dauphine SL, Maki BE. Measuring balance in the elderly: validation of an instrument. *Canadian Journal of Public Health.* 1992: 83: 7-11.

6. Boyce W, Gowland C, Rosenbaum P, et al. Gross Motor Performance Measure for Children with Cerebral Palsy: Study Design and Preliminary Findings. *Canadian Journal of Public Health* 1992: 83 (2): S34-S40.

D.11. Movement Assessment of Infants (MAI)

1. Chandler LS, Andrew MS, Swanson MW. *Movement Assessment of Infants - a Manual.* Rolling Bay, WA. 98061: P.O. Box 4631; 1980.

2. Campbell SK. Movement Assessment of Infants: an evaluation. *Physical and Occupational Therapy in Pediatrics* 1982: 1 (4): 53-57.

3. Deitz JC, Crowe TK, Harris SR. Relationship between infant neuromotor assessment and preschool motor measures. *Phys Ther* 1987: 67 (1): 14-17.

4. Hayley SM, Harris SR, Tada WL, Swanson MS. Item reliability of Movement Assessment of Infants. *Physical and Occupational Therapy in Pediatrics* 1986: 6 (1): 21-29.

5. Harris SR, Swanson MW, Andrews MS, et al. Predictive validity of the movement assessment of infants. *J Dev Behav Pediatr* 1984: 5: 336-343.

6.   Lydic JS, Short MA, Nelson DI. Comparison of two scales for assessing motor development in infants with Down's syndrome. *The Occupational Therapy Journal of Research* 1983: 3 (4): 213-221.

7.   Harris SR. Early detection of cerebral palsy: sensitivity and specificity of two motor assessment tools. *J Perinatol* 1987: 7 (1): 11-15.

8.   Harris SR. Early neuromotor predictor of cerebral palsy in low-weight infants. *Dev Med Child Neurol* 1987: 29: 508-519.

Other Reading

Paban M, Piper MC. Early predictors of one year neurodevelopmental outcome for "at risk" infants. *Physical and Occupational Therapy in Pediatrics* 1987: 7 (3): 17-34.

Palisano RJ. Review of research on reliability and validity of the Movement Assessment of Infants. *Pediatric Physical Therapy* 1989: 1 (4): 167-172.

Schneider JW, Lee W, Chasnoff IJ. Field testing of the movement assessment of infants. *Phys Ther* 1988: 68 (3): 321-327.

Swanson MW, Bennett FC, Shy KK, Whitfield MF. Identification of neurodevelopmental abnormality at four and eight months by the movement assessment of infants. *Dev Med Child Neurol* 1992: 34 (4): 321-338.

D.12. Pediatric Evaluation of Disability Inventory (PEDI)

1.   Haley SM, Coster WJ, Ludlow LH, Haltiwanger JT, Andrellos PJ. *Pediatric Evaluation of Disability Inventory (PEDI). Development, Standardization and Administration Manual* 1992.

2.   Feldman AB, Haley SM, Coryell J. Concurrent and construct validity of the Pediatric Evaluation of Disability Inventory. *Phys Ther* 1990:70(10):602-610.

REFERENCES FOR PART IV

1.   Gonnella C. Our new venture. *Arch Phys Med Rehabil* 1992: 73: s1-s2.

2.   Issues and Recommendations from Proceedings of National Workshop on Patient Outcome Measures. *Don Mills, Toronto: Hospital Medical Records Institute 1991.*

3.   World Health Organization (WHO) . International classification of impairments, disabilities and handicaps. A manual of classification relating to the consequences of disease. Geneva: *World Health Organization* 1980.

4.   Johnston MV, Keith RA, Hinderer SR. Measurement standards for interdisciplinary medical rehabilitation. *Arch Phys Med Rehabil* 1992: 73: s3-s23.

5.   Gowland C, Stratford P, Ward M, et al. Measuring physical impairment and disability with the Chedoke-McMaster Stroke Assessment. *Stroke* 1993: 24 (1): 58-63.

6.   Palisano RJ, Haley SM, Brown DA. Goal attainment scaling as a measure of change in infants with motor delays. *Phys Ther* 1992: 72 (6): 432-437.

7.   Malec JF, Smigielski JS, DePompolo RW. Goal attainment scaling and outcome measurement in postacute brain injury rehabilitation. *Arch Phys Med Rehabil* 1991: 72: 138-143.

8.   Ottenbacher KJ, Cusick A. Goal attainment scaling as a method of clinical service evaluation. *AJOT* 1990: 44 (6): 519-527.

9.   Hayley SM, Baryza MJ, Lewin MJ, Cioffi MI. Sensorimotor dysfunction in children with brain injury: development of a data base for evaluation research. *Physical and Occupational Therapy in Pediatrics* 1991: 11 (3): 1-26.

10. State University of New York at Buffalo Department of Rehabilitation Medicine. *Guide for use of the Uniform Data Set for Medical Rehabilitation including the Functional Independence Measure (FIM)* 1990.

INDEX